BUT SERIOUSLY.

Wh KNEW?

BUT SERIOUSLY,

WHO OHO

KNEW?

MY CANCER *and other bits* STORY

MELANIE GREEN

FIRST EDITION

Book design by Publishing Push

ISBNs:
Paperback: 978-1-80227-579-7
eBook: 978-1-80227-580-3

www.melaniegreenauthor.co.uk

Cheers to Big G, Lauren and Kieron, and to having very
inappropriate humour in the darkest of times.
Love you zillions xxx

Contents

A Letter to Myself Before Cancer

Dear Mel (BC),

Chill your beans honey, don't sweat the small stuff. It doesn't matter about the ironing. It doesn't matter about the dust. It doesn't matter about the weeds and the long grass. It doesn't matter…what matters is family, friends, and doing things that make you happy.

Appreciate nature as it is – the birds singing, the blue sky, the green grass – they won't get any sweeter, bluer or greener, even though after the diagnosis you think they will!

Blissful ignorance and believing it will never happen to you is great but unfortunately it *will* happen to you.

One day you are really going to question the meaning of life and try to answer 'why me?' – not sure you'll ever know the answer, no matter how hard you look, or how many people you ask!

Life really is too short: stop waiting for it to begin, be proactive and make it happen. Stop saying 'one day' – make it *today*. Make sure you appreciate the small things in life. Stop trying to have, get, be…more – YOU ARE ENOUGH.

Well done for being a clumsy clot as one day it will save your life. Stop wasting time on people who don't go the extra mile for you. One day you will see who your true, and real, friends are.

Lots of Love x

1. Well, I Guess I Should Just Get on and Write!

Everyone's story is unique. That's what makes us special. One story is not more important than another, just different. We all live with whatever comes our way. Some of us believe in fate, some of us believe that we determine our own destiny, some of us believe a bit of both…that's me! I never really thought my story was that interesting as it is my normal. But when I've spoken to friends, colleagues, and even strangers, they seem to want to know more. From adoption, marriage, divorce, another marriage, children and miscarriage; to jobs, university, cancer and aliens living in my head, just to mention a few 'highlights'! So here goes…

Fifty (now 52 – it took me a while to finish writing this)! Firstly WTF…secondly how on earth…and thirdly thank God for that!

I'm sure it's a common feeling when you reach this ripe old age, but how the hell am I 50? Mentally I barely feel 25 but then my body sometimes feels 70, so I guess I should be happy I'm somewhere in the middle. But 50!? I've always wanted to celebrate every birthday (they are all special, right?)…apart from my 23rd when I had a meltdown realising I was nearer to 25 than 20, married with one child and another on the way…but age is just a number and I've invariably thought it's a privilege to be getting older as not everyone gets the chance. Being diagnosed with breast cancer just after my 48th birthday has made this even more of a reality and I just want to share my story. Not just about cancer, but some other 'exciting' moments and stories that have influenced or changed me in my 50 years on earth. I'm using this book to reflect, look back, maybe as a bit of self-analysis, to ask myself lots of questions, but probably to get very few answers.

I'm fairly sure there will be lots of jumping about with no chronological order, as I'm not the most structured when I write – or in life. I don't edit or read as I go and then I try really hard not to change anything apart from spellings and grammar afterwards. So, these are my unfiltered thoughts and feelings flowing straight on to the page as a stream of consciousness. I've written three blogs in the past – two that included general ponderings and life BC, and the other about my cancer story. I am planning on using these as a basis for this book, while filling in some blanks, adding other life bits and we'll see where it takes me. You will find that any excerpts taken straight from the blogs are dated with when they were written, as well as being in italics and in a box, which hopefully will make this a bit easier to navigate! Of course, I couldn't leave them as they were and had to add bits as I went through them – you will find these added extras in square brackets [!]. I'll try to keep the chapters short because if you are anything like me and you are reading this in bed, you won't be able to stop in the middle of a chapter...no matter how tired you are, and then you'll have to re-read the last few pages in the morning! Although, obviously, please feel free to find it an 'unputdownable' book!

This is a personal story and therefore is likely to offend at times as I can be terribly inappropriate, but then I guess it's up to you whether you continue to read. I promise to be very honest and open and wear my heart on my sleeve (which is my natural way to be), so this book is my story, warts and all.

And I apologise in advance for the swearing...

So, a little about me, and mine. I'm Melanie (Mel to newly introduced people as when I get nervous, I can't say my name without too many LLLLs!). I'm married to Big G (Graham) and we have three children between us – Lauren, Kieron and Kirstie. I'm not sure what else to tell you at this stage, except that I can guarantee you will find out more than you want to know about my bodily functions as we go through this (it gets a bit TMI)!

2. 'I'm Afraid it's Cancer'

This seems the obvious place to start. The paragraphs below are from a blog post that seemed to touch so many people's hearts (thank you for every message I've had). It cemented both my love for writing, and also for sharing my experiences with anyone who wanted to 'listen'. Cancer and all its 'special joys' really came as a surprise to me. I knew nothing about it – cancer was cancer and chemo was chemo. But seriously, who fucking knew (hence the book title!)? There's a lot that I didn't know, and if it wasn't for this book, I hope you never have to know either – I've also added a handy cheat sheet at the end to help with the terminology. I had no idea how many different types there were of both cancer and chemotherapy, and even when we are just talking about breast cancer, how there could be so many different variations and so many different ways this could go. I had no idea of the side effects I would have and even the booklet they give you doesn't list them all. But then again, I guess people would run away screaming if they really knew what was potentially in store, and also everyone experiences their story differently so there is no way of knowing whether you would get each and every side effect, or none at all!

31st July 2018 –
On the 1st of every month, Lauren and I receive a text [from the CoppaFeel! Breast Cancer charity (this is me writing now, in the present day, hi!)] _to remind us to check our boobs. If we are together, we laugh as they come through at the same time and also chuckle at the poem used to encourage us to get checking ourselves. But did we ever check? Did we heck as like!_ [I do now!] _But I did find my_

3

lump anyway, even though I'm not quite old enough to start having mammograms, and here is how!

Big G can never moan at me for being a clumsy clot again as falling over most definitely saved my life...

Rewind back to the end of April 2018 and Lauren had just bought a new flat. We were there trying to get it sorted and I got my foot caught in the cord of a venetian blind. Imagine Eddie the Eagle flying through the air but ending with a face plant on the floor and that was me! Lauren actually thought I was dead for a few seconds as I wasn't moving and she thought I'd banged my head on a storage heater, which was filled with concrete. Through tears, and laughter, I exclaimed, 'I think I've just popped my boob' and both knees started to swell before our eyes.

I have fallen over many times over the years...hence Big G having a bit of an issue with my clumsiness. One spectacular fall left me with the biggest black eye, well half a face, having gone arse over tit. After one too many sherbets (shock I know!) I clearly forgot I'd got arms, resulting in my face landing on the pavement. A week or two later, still with concussion and the most colourful face, we went away for the weekend. I joked that I was going to flinch every time Big G came near me, but then he pointed out that when I laughed and said I was joking, people may still not believe me...and would think that I was probably too scared of him to tell the truth. But I swear, we had great service everywhere we went – now did they feel sorry for me, or were they worried that he may get nifty with his fists if they didn't give us those extra pots of guacamole and salsa for our nachos?!

Just to add, having Game as my surname also caused some name calling...on the game, game for a laugh, game for anything, two out of three may be correct – I will leave you to decide which ones! Kids are flipping horrid, aren't they? Oh, that's just made me think of a story – see I told you I would jump about a bit (and digress)! When I say 'they' are horrid, I was one of 'them'...not the worst and I wouldn't call myself a bully but I remember at junior school telling one girl to 'piss off' just as the head teacher walked into the hall...oops. I was marched to the office for a lecture, where I was told I should know better than to swear as both of my parents were (at the time) teachers! Now I have no idea why this should have made a difference but I couldn't vent my indignation when I got home or I would have had to tell Mum and Dad what I'd done – and then I would definitely have been in a whole heap of trouble. I probably even will be now for swearing, sorry Mum!

31st July 2018 –
    Who knew falling over could cause such a bruise inside! So, I left it a week or so before going to the doctors as they were only going to tell me not to be ridiculous, and of course the lump was the result of the fall. Er wrong,
    'We need to refer you to the breast clinic Mrs Green but it doesn't mean it's cancer.'

5

I put my arms above my head when I got home that night and looked at my boob – it was only by turning to the side that I could see the large indentation underneath. I know this is a sign of cancer but in all honesty, I wouldn't have ever noticed this unless I checked myself thoroughly which, as you know already, I didn't! Not that I would have known to look in the mirror with my arms up even if I did check myself – please make sure you add this to your monthly checking routine.

31st July 2018 –
    ...and then sent me along for a mammogram and ultrasound scan [25th May 2018].
    For those of you that have had the pleasure of a mammogram you will know the joy...squeezing F cup boobs down to the size of AA, whilst getting the stomach-fat out of the way of the machine – nothing to be embarrassed about here! Then off for the ultrasound scan where I expected them to laugh at me again as this was just a bruise. Er wrong again,
    'We'll just put a little needle in to take a small biopsy Mrs Green' and so he took a core biopsy as I lay on the bed and squeezed the poor nurse's hand so hard, I'm surprised she didn't join me in crying! The process didn't really hurt, due to the local anaesthetic, but the realisation was beginning to hit that maybe this wasn't just a bruise. The bloody doctor who was stroking my arm sympathetically didn't help this thought process either! Who knew that if they suspect you have cancer, everyone becomes so kind and gentle – even receptionists at the doctor's surgery!

After the biopsy we spoke to the consultant who said it was a 50/50 chance of being cancer. Now that I look back, I think they knew it was 100% cancer at the time but they needed to know what type it was before telling me. Without this information they wouldn't have been able to tell me a treatment plan and I would have been full of questions without them knowing all of the answers.

31st July 2018 –
Then a wait of ten days, until Monday 4th June 2018, for the results... during which I thought the 'not knowing' was the worst thing in the world – turns out that is total bollocks and the 'knowing' is actually a zillion times worse when it's not good news.

Throughout this time there were only five people who knew that I was having tests – Big G, Kerstey [my bestie] and her hubby, my boss and another work friend. After all, why on earth would I tell my family and worry them to death when there was absolutely nothing to worry about. This thought was confounded by the fact that a psychic had told me, admittedly many years before, that I would never have cancer – think it's time for me to claim a refund!

There were many times in this 10-day period that I went into meltdown – having to face the reality of my mortality. I had to put a brave face on for my birthday, told numerous lies about where I was, took time off work because I couldn't hold it together, and my sister Bryony (Bry) was convinced I was being really off with her because I didn't seem like myself (and was clearly doing a shitty job at lying). It didn't make it any easier that it was also Dad's birthday during this time. I was so evasive when Bry was trying to make arrangements that she thought I didn't care. In reality I was just scared that I couldn't keep up the smiling pretence act for more than half an hour at a time, so avoiding everyone was easier!

I also made many inappropriate comments when we went out with Kerstey and Nic [Kerstey's husband] during this time, playing on the fact they needed to be nice to me as I may be dying (Big G was not impressed with these jokes)! Being inappropriate helped me deal with the stress and these were some of the only people in the world that knew what was going on at that moment. The night before I was getting my results I drank copious amounts of wine with Kerstey and there were many, many tears – how on earth could I tell my kids if it was cancer? I wasn't ready to die, I wasn't ready to leave my beautiful family, they needed me and I needed them – more than ever now.

31st July 2018 –

Fast-forward to 4pm on that dreaded Monday afternoon [4th June 2018] and I'd just told Big G on the way to the hospital that I had a very good feeling and everything was going to be fine. Not sure who I was trying to convince but I think he believed me for a few minutes. The waiting room in the breast clinic emptied out, as people were called through for their appointments, and Big G said 'And then there was one'. In hindsight I still wonder if we had an appointment at the end of the day so anyone there for initial tests wouldn't be scared if they heard me cry/scream/howl once the guillotine dropped. At this point we were shepherded into a room and the nurse kept busy around us making small talk and tidying everything in sight. Eventually, she left and the consultant arrived. As soon as we saw him walk in with someone else, we looked at each other and knew, we just felt it, that this was not going to be good news – it doesn't take two people to tell you that you have been wasting their time and to go away and have a good life.

'I'm afraid it's cancer'.

I told them they had the wrong script, that this one wasn't meant for me, but they just looked sympathetically at me and reassured me that they hadn't got it wrong...not the type of reassurance I wanted at this point!

I'm not sure I can tell you what was actually said, just lots of words, none of them good, none of them making any sense, but...there was talk of cure and not 'just' prolonging life and so this is what I clung on to. There were many emotions...fear, but I would think that is a fairly obvious one; guilt, because of what I was about to put my loved ones through; and relief, because I hadn't been making a mountain out of a molehill. I'd had the previous week off work as my brain wouldn't function, not knowing if I was being overly dramatic – well that relief was a stupid emotion as now I would rather have been laughed at for being a lightweight and dramatic than having to do this – but the relief was real!

When you hear those fateful words, no matter what else is said, it feels like a death-sentence. The world speeds up, the world slows down, the world falls off its axis. What the hell? This cannot possibly be happening – not to me. I'm a good person, I'm a mother, a wife, a daughter, a sister, an auntie – I can't have cancer.

Telling my loved ones that I had cancer was one of the hardest things I've ever had to do. As a mother you are meant to protect your family – not devastate them with one sentence. From the hospital, I went straight to Bryony's so that I could 'practise' on her first. After dropping the news on her, I went to the toilet and when I came back in the room Big G and her were talking in hushed voices – oh no, it had already started...the pity, the fear, the worry. Then I had to tell Lauren and Kieron. I wanted to tell them together but Kieron was at the gym when Lauren got home from work and she knew something was very wrong. I couldn't pretend so I told her. It took ages for Kieron to come back – he told me later that he'd had a feeling something was wrong as he had previously heard me and Big G talking about a hospital appointment. So, he went to a mate's house after the gym as I was apparently acting a bit strange before he had left the house. I sat with them both on my bed and after the tears came the inappropriate jokes, thank goodness, and then we just got on with it. Lauren and I had an 'oh no' moment a few weeks later – I'd always joked about her writing to '60-minute makeover' but we never had an emotional story to tell – now we had a story but the show wasn't on TV anymore, gutted! I had to wait a week to tell Mum and Dad as Mum was away with my aunt. Mum burst into tears; Dad collapsed on the floor. One of the worst things imaginable had come into our lives and somehow, someway, we needed to get through it – together.

31st July 2018 –

My breast cancer diagnosis is carcinoma of the right breast – locally advanced grade 3 invasive ductal cancer, ER+ (oestrogen receptor positive – approx. 70% of breast cancers are ER+) and HER2+ (progesterone positive with human epidermal growth factor which is a protein that affects the growth of the cancer cells – this is the one that makes it aggressive – affecting approx. 20% of breast cancer patients). This means I need to have eight sessions of chemotherapy (two different types – the first four sessions being FEC-T – Fluorouracil, Epirubicin, Cyclophosphamide and Docetaxel; with the next four sessions being Pertuzumab, Trastuzumab, and Docetaxel – and no, I don't know what any of those mean!); this will be followed by surgery (not sure if that will consist of a lumpectomy or a full mastectomy), and then radiotherapy, hormone therapy, and Herceptin injections which help prevent the cancer coming back. Since my diagnosis I have had confirmation that the cancer has not spread – when I got that news I wanted to dance and celebrate. This is a victory, but it still seems weird celebrating that you have cancer, but it's not as bad as it could be!

I can't work during the chemo because of the risk of infection, which is very high due to working in a college environment. This has completely rocked my world, and obviously those around me. People keep saying I'm brave the way I am facing it – I don't feel brave, I feel fucking terrified, but what choice do I have. I want to grow old, I want *to hold my grandchildren (no pressure kids), I want to travel and see the world, I want to drink hot chocolate with Big G whilst rocking in a chair (either because I'm sitting on a rocking chair or because I'm just bloody old), I want to do soooo many things – so I CAN'T let this beat me, I WON'T let this beat me. Come on cancer – do your fucking worst.*

Well, I definitely put up a good fight. Although, I am a bit wary about using terms like 'fighting', 'being a warrior', etc., as to me it makes it seem like anyone who has died from this hideous illness did not try to live and fight hard enough, and that's clearly a ridiculous statement. Everyone uses the language that suits them whilst in their own version of the cancer story, as they should. I just don't personally like to consider myself a warrior or that I fought harder than anyone else. I class myself as lucky, and hopefully will not have to endure it, or be lucky, again.

I consciously didn't Google too much after I was initially diagnosed, although I have to admit that I definitely did a bit! I stopped myself most of the time because it scared the bejesus out of me. I tried, where possible, to wait until I was told what I needed to know rather than jumping the gun and predicting my outcome. I'm sure a lot of people ask a lot more questions than I did…but I just did as I was told, went where I was told to go, 'put your boob in here', 'put your arms in there', etc. The not knowing led to some confusion further down the line but that's just how I coped with it. You have no idea how to react in the moment and there is no instruction manual to tell you how to feel. You just have to cope with it in the best way you can at the time. There is no right way; there is no wrong way; there is just your way.

3. Winning at Cancer!

31st July 2018 –
> *Maybe a weird one, but how do you win at cancer??!*

I posted this blog post on a Facebook group I follow and got quite a lot of negative comments, which shows they clearly didn't actually read the post! Just to clarify…'win at cancer' in this case doesn't mean being given the all clear as you will see if you keep reading!

31st July 2018 –
> *This question came up when I was wig shopping with Lauren not long after my diagnosis* [I actually only wore the wig once as I felt a bit silly with it on for some reason. I preferred to wear a scarf, less scratchy and less hot!]. *Whilst we were shopping, another lady was there looking at the wigs and seemed quite upset. Me being me, tried to make light of the situation and said, 'At least you can be who you want to be'.*
>
> *To which she replied sadly, 'But it's the reason I'm doing this'.*
> *'Me too', was my response.*
> *She then went on to tell me that she was 'triple negative'…*
> *'Er, I've got some positive bits', was my reply. I purposely walked away at this point as I didn't want to 'talk' cancer, and I certainly didn't want to engage further and have a cancer buddy.*
>
> *But she clearly knew more about this cancer jargon than I did (I told you I didn't ask enough questions!) but it got me wondering about her diagnosis and whether it was worse or better than mine – not that this matters a jot but hey, that's how my mind works. So, which is winning…?*
> *If you have 'more/worse' breast cancer or 'less serious' breast cancer.*

Let me explain my reasoning...I compared it to childbirth. If you have a labour of seventy-two hours, hell on earth that results in an emergency caesarean, then you win when discussing it with other mothers. You also win if you give birth in twenty minutes, with no pain relief and hardly break into a sweat. But...if you have a

'normal' twelve-hour labour, use gas and air and any other pain relief offered, then

you most certainly do not win. You are average, nondescript, boring! And don't we all try to win with our nearest and dearest? I can't think of many times that I have said I've got a cold without Big G saying he has flu, or a bad back without him saying he can hardly walk. And I'm sure we have all complained about having a bad night and the response being, 'Well I only had twenty minutes sleep all night!'

Is it the same with cancer? If you have a 'little' cancer, are you winning? Or are you only winning if you are terminal?

And here's one of the inappropriate moments I warned you about...I had to have a clip fitted in the tumour so that if the chemo reduced the size, the surgeon would still know the area to remove during surgery. While Lauren and I were waiting in the reception area, a lady kept crying, clearly worried about being there. The nurse told me that the rest of the people there that day were recalls from routine mammograms where they had either found something that needed looking in to, or they needed a repeat mammogram as they couldn't read the results clearly. When I got back to Lauren in the waiting room, I said, 'Well I'm winning today – these people don't even know if they have cancer or not!'

Heartless maybe, Ok definitely, but you deal with stuff in whichever way gets you through.

My only hope, obvious I'm sure, is that I WIN at beating this shit and become cancer free...I'm sure that will really mean I'm winning, even if it does just come down to sheer luck.

And there is the language again...words like winning, losing, fighting. But it doesn't always come down to how well we fight, or how strong we think we are compared to our opponent. Some of us just swing a lucky punch, hit the vulnerable spot and send cancer flying across the ring, whereas some of us go for the full twelve rounds and lose on a technicality, a corrupt referee, or another cancer illegally jumps in the ring to help his mate out so it's two against one!

4. Hair Loss and Bird Poo

31st July 2018 –
> When I was diagnosed, my oncology nurse Rachel explained about the side effects that may occur with the chemotherapy – hair loss being one of them. My sister came to the first oncology appointment with me and Big G so she could take notes and ask the questions we forgot about. She asked about using a cold cap to help prevent hair loss (my kids and her had been discussing this thinking that I would really struggle with losing my hair) but we were told that with the type of chemo I would be having it would not help. On being told that the 'cold' is -5 degrees I was kind of relieved that I didn't need to even think about this – as you will see through out these posts, I am a complete wimp and therefore do not feel the need to subject myself to anymore pain, or fear, than is absolutely necessary – no theme parks or scary films for me, not even Crimewatch thank you very much.

I've always been quite adventurous with my hair, colouring and perming it from the age of 13. I trained as a hairdresser when Kieron started school and I was 28. I really wanted to do it when I left school but it didn't pay enough so I went to work in a bank – thinking that I was being clever and I would be able to get a staff mortgage. Finding out, at 16, that I would have to wait until I was 23 before that could happen meant I only lasted at the bank for a year and a half! I digress (shock)…but the minute I started the hairdressing course, the colours and styles became more extreme – even though I was a mother of two and I'm sure other people thought I should have acted my age! However, looking back now, 28 is still very young so I'm glad I went a bit wild! I don't think losing my hair was as much of an issue for me as it was for those around me. You often hear of people, especially women, finding that losing their hair is the worst thing about cancer as it can feel like you are losing your identity. Luckily most of the time I have no idea what my 'identity' is! Because the hair loss wasn't an issue, I wasn't at all prepared for the tears and emotions that came whilst drinking a vat of wine when I had my hair cut in preparation for it.

> 31st July 2018 –
> The weekend before my first chemo session my sister-in-law, Sandra, cut my hair really short, and coloured it, so that the shock wouldn't be so great once I started losing it. I went for a darker shade than normal, knowing that the grey wouldn't have time to come through...always a bonus! I actually found this process more distressing than when my hair started to fall out but I think this was probably more to do with the fear about what was coming.
> Rachel had told me that my body hair would probably not go until the second type of chemo, so imagine my surprise when a week and a half after my first chemo session I had a handful of fanwah hair whilst having a shower. Surprise but also a bit of delight – no more having to shave the ever-greying pubes! Further delight was the loss of underarm hair, and the slowing down of leg hair growth...another bonus!

With the second group of chemo (the last four sessions), I lost all of my body hair – eyebrows, eyelashes, nostrils, legs and arms – smooth like a baby's bottom! After finishing chemo, and as hairy as ever (even a few more chin ones due to age and added hormones/menopause), I joke…probably inappropriately…that another quick blast of chemo would be fab thank you very much. Less of a task than shaving, and less painful than waxing – actually not less painful but it was rather nice not having hairy legs etc. Not that I ended up going out, during the last few months of having chemo, to show my smooth legs and hairless armpits off to anyone!

> 31st July 2018 –
> *Two days later, just under two weeks since starting chemo, the pain started! Who knew that losing your hair could be soooo painful? My whole scalp felt incredibly bruised and I couldn't bear to touch my hair at all. By three o'clock the next morning I just had to get up as just lying on the pillow was killing me. So, Google to the rescue and the answer was to shave the bugger off. To be honest it was already coming out in handfuls anyway so I felt I was only losing a few extra days of having hair. Apparently, the chemo causes the hair follicles to become inflamed so any movement of the hair is painful which I found out the hard way.*

Even after all of my hair had gone my scalp remained really painful and sensitive – a light shower of rain was excruciating.

> 31st July 2018 –
> *Lauren set to it with the clippers, which I'm sure was quite surreal for her but she volunteered so I didn't feel too bad that she had to do such a momentous thing. Kieron was about as well and they were both surprised at how 'normal' I looked without hair – he even said I reminded him of Amber Rose, a model – a little chuffed!*

In reality I looked like one of the Mitchell brothers from Eastenders – so Big G was Phil and I was Grant, obviously as Grant is the better looking one! Lauren said I looked like a boiled egg – ever the confidence booster!! Haha!

> 31st July 2018 –
> *Big G then wet shaved it for me, not the most pleasant experience as it felt like it was ripping the remaining hair out – new respect for him as he has to shave off the little he has left every few days and it*

Three years on and it's bloody grey, in dreadful condition and definitely curlier than it was!

When I was hairdressing, I had the 'privilege' of shaving a couple of customers' hair when they started losing it because of cancer treatment. It was a very upsetting experience but I was so happy that I could provide a safe environment where they felt comfortable (having Charlie's head, our gorgeous Labradoodle, resting on their laps seemed to calm them) and free to cry, not something they felt they could do in a salon. I couldn't charge for this 'service' so I asked them to donate something to charity as they both wanted to pay. I did the same when I styled someone's hair to attend a loved one's funeral – how can you profit from such horrendous times?

31st July 2018 –

Luckily, I have an ok shaped head, not that I think I will have the confidence to leave the house au naturel, but I did discover a new birthmark on the back of my head. But then came the mystery...a dirty brown stain along the top of my head that resembled a massive streak of bird poo! A birthmark we all thought initially, then...could it have been the hair dye but that had happened too many weeks, and hair washes, before. But then Lauren came up with the solution – suntan! It was where I had my parting so this part of my scalp had had many years of sun. The only problem is I'm not allowed to sit in the sun so the chance of getting the rest of my scalp to match anytime soon is fairly remote – so my bird poo and I are stuck with each other!

Thankfully the tan faded after a while, and my hair stopped growing, so I was left with a white, shiny scalp and no shaving. It's remarkable how quickly you can shower and get out of the house when you don't have to do your hair, just wash and shine – that is until chemo really took its toll and then showering became a bit of an event, which usually involved a lie down before attempting to get dressed, and not much going out! It didn't bother me deeply about having no hair, but I never got used to the staring. This meant I didn't leave the scarf off until I had a shadow of hair – but that still felt quite momentous and everyone still bloody stared.

5. Who Knew It Would Be Poo That Would Floor Me?

> 3rd August 2018 –
>
> Chemotherapy is basically a mixture of poisons that aim to kill all the bad cancer cells, but unfortunately it affects all the good ones too. I have just had session number three and each treatment seems to have brought different side effects – here is an update so far...
>
> 18th June 2018 – 1st Chemo
>
> Fear of the unknown, expecting the worst, still in a very surreal world believing this cannot possibly be happening to me, they've got it wrong – made even more surreal that they had written Michelle Green on my appointment card!! The receptionist assured me that it was me, and not Michelle that should be there, but I could only imagine Michelle sitting at home thinking that she was fine and dandy, and I was going to have her treatment by mistake – unfortunately it was just a clerical error!
>
> I had many tears after the cannula was put in but when the nurse started administering the chemo I think a calmness just came over me, knowing that this had to happen to cure me of this hideous disease. A few hours later it was time to go home with the tiniest plaster on the back of my hand – it didn't really represent the horror of the day!

I had four different types of chemotherapy for the first four sessions (FEC-T: Fluorouracil, Epirubicin, Cyclophosphamide, and Docetaxel). They had to be given very slowly, by hand, through the cannula. This took a good couple of hours and therefore involved fairly intimate conversations with whichever nurse was sitting by my knee, administering the drugs, for the duration...with the odd inappropriate comment thrown in by Big G! The oncology nurses were all amazing. I never felt rushed; I never felt pressured to put on a brave face – even when I was being a baby about having the sticky pad pulled off that kept the cannula in place! They were smiley, genuine and oh-so-caring. You would expect a cancer centre to be a miserable, depressing place but that is so far off the mark. Luckily the Woolverstone Day Unit at Ipswich Hospital is bright and modern after a makeover a few years ago (2016), which also added to the feeling of calm and well-being. After the first session, the nurse explained that the Epirubicin would turn my wee red…. I probably shouldn't have got so excited when I went to the loo and she was right! It was a bit like when you have a wee after eating asparagus and it smells funny – schoolgirl humour! I left armed with a bunch of pills – anti-sickness, steroids and antibiotics – luckily, she wrote on each packet when I needed to take them as my head was in a complete spin and I still wasn't taking much in!

> 3rd August 2018 –
> Once I left the hospital, a dry mouth and sick feeling were almost instant. This was kind of a blessing as I'm rubbish at drinking water and this is required to fight off infections. A couple of mouth ulcers erupted but these soon disappeared when I started my course of antibiotics. I have to take these for ten days at the most vulnerable time for infections – this is the main thing the nurses/doctors warn you about. Food and people being the things to watch out for. I had no idea about these things – such a steep learning curve! I love to learn, hence doing a degree in my 40's, but I really never wanted to know so much about cancer, its treatment and its treats!

It was a bit like being pregnant with the things you are not allowed to eat, although I was pregnant a long time ago so the guidelines are stricter now – I even got the taste for lager when I was pregnant with Kieron, haha, but I only had the occasional one…promise! The foods to avoid when having chemotherapy include: meats/salads etc.

from the deli counter, unpasteurised milk and other dairy products, live yogurts, soft/unpasteurised/blue cheeses, smoked fish, pâté, unwashed fruit and vegetables, raw fish and shellfish. You also need to ensure all meat and eggs are cooked thoroughly – so all a bit rubbish really! It's amazing how quickly you crave a rare steak and a soft-boiled egg when you can't have them.

3rd August 2018 –
   On the whole I breezed through the first treatment (apart from the hair loss pain) but...
9th July – 2nd Chemo
   Still fear but no tears this time – I'm sooo brave!! Lol A dry mouth but no ulcers this time. Well, this is easy-peasy...er NOT! So maybe too much information but Thursday eve (three days in) and I feel like I need the loo. OMG the pain. Suddenly I am so constipated and it feels like I am trying to shit a brick. We were staying at Priory Park (we have a lodge there) and so Big G went home to get me some Dulcolax, which is a miracle cure. Wrong...did nothing for me. Spent the night literally screaming in pain, trying to soak in the smallest bath in the world to soften everything up – nothing worked. Friday morning Big G went to the chemist to get me suppositories, which also didn't work very well. I don't think I have ever felt pain like it – possibly when I gave birth but at least you get a bundle of joy at the end of it! Although if I could have got the poo out, I think I would have cuddled it! Eventually after more suppositories and laxatives, and oh so many tears and lots of screams, I had some relief. As you can imagine, this left me with several piles so the next few days were very painful and involved me sitting on a pillow!

In hindsight I should have gone to the hospital but being very 'British', I didn't like to make a fuss – especially about poo! As I hadn't slept much that night, I tried to get a few hours in the afternoon whilst waiting for the meds to kick in.

'Call me if you need me' said Big G as he went to sit in the lounge. Another 'try' on the loo had me screaming his name – not sure what I expected him to do but I felt I needed his company. No answer, no rushing to soothe me…where was he? Fast asleep on the bloody sofa! I tried to find the funny side of this, until it happened again an hour later! I can't imagine what the neighbours thought; I must have sounded like I was being beaten up with all the screaming and crying.

> 3rd August 2018 –
>   Afterwards I knew I could not possibly go through this again, so I picked up a massive prescription bundle (Laxido and Senokot) from the doctor ready for chemo session number three.
>   Oh, and I also had a bit of incontinence! Why-oh-why: isn't having no hair, piles, and constipation enough? No? Why not make me pee myself while just making the bed in the morning!!

The incontinence is still an issue occasionally but is so much better, thank goodness. I just have to remember not to leave it too late before going to the loo, or I have to stand/sit still until I have the courage to move…hooray for Tena Lady! I wonder why they don't give medication to prevent constipation as a matter of course when you are starting chemo, but some people go the other way and have diarrhoea so I guess it's the 'luck' of the draw!

> 3rd August 2018 –
> 30th July – 3rd Chemo
>   Well, you can only imagine how nervous and anxious I was about this one after 'shit saga'. But I have been popping the laxatives, drinking the softeners, and so far, so good (it is now Friday evening so hopefully over the worst – apparently it is the mix of anti-sickness and chemo that causes the constipation). Felt a little sicky, and definitely a bit bleugh for a few days but feeling more myself today, no siesta needed – and even looking forward to the tapas feast that Big G is preparing for tea! So hopefully I am in for a couple of good weeks before chemo session number four!

6. Edge of Panic

22nd August 2018 –

On Monday, 20th Aug, I had my 4th chemo session – the same drugs as the last three sessions. So why when Big G asked me how I was, before we left for the hospital, did I respond by saying 'I'm on the edge of panic'? This feeling had been with me most of Sunday and by Monday (the day of my chemo appointment) I was wondering if I could really put myself through this again. I obviously knew I had no choice as the treatment is working (as far as I'm aware) so there is no question of me not continuing but I was suddenly so scared and so close to a panic attack.

After my last blog post I had a great weekend. On the Saturday, the week before, (11th August) Big G and I walked down to the seafront and even had a glass of wine! Yes, I can have a glass when I fancy it, I checked with the consultant...his reply was 'Yes you can, but most women don't!' Oh, that will be just me then!

Once I got onto the fifth session, a month or so after this, I realised what he meant – *even I* didn't fancy wine, which shows how rubbish I felt!

22rd August 2018 –

Then the next day (12th August), I was still feeling really good so I cleaned the house – maybe I wasn't feeling good at all as cleaning is not my normal 'go to' activity as many friends will testify!! But looking back I think I maybe did too much as by the Monday morning I was on my arse. I felt horrid, light headed, and just totally drained. So, I spent the next four or five days on the sofa, which sounds heaven but really is not. It was a boiling hot week and my baldhead kept sticking to the leather sofa...why would anyone buy a leather sofa, never again! Could this have been the reason for my sudden, and totally overwhelming panic? Or could it be that I knew this was the last of this mix of drugs and the next four chemo sessions will consist of new drugs that I have no idea how I will react to?

On arriving at hospital on Monday, I was told that my blood test (done on Saturday) had come back showing my white blood count was very low so they may have to delay chemo – I was kind of relieved but also pee'd off that I was going to have to go through these feelings again in another few days. But after another blood test, the count had gone up so in the chemo drugs went. I'm feeling relatively ok, so clearly no need to panic – just going to be a bit more sensible this time and let Big G do the cleaning!!!

Just a quick, and I think quite amusing, fact to lighten the mood... who knew that when you have chemo they advise you use a condom for the first few days after each session as the chemotherapy drugs can be transferred to your partner through either seminal or vaginal fluid? To be honest, hanky-panky is the furthest thing from my mind straight after chemo – soz Big G!

7. If You Don't Laugh, You'll Cry!

5th September 2018 –
> *Clearly, I have done something wrong in my life! Why else would cancer alone not be enough?! Let's throw a bit of tinnitus and shingles in!*

If only I knew when I wrote this how true that statement was. I really must have been a massive bitch…there is so much more to come in this story – we haven't even scratched the surface yet!

5th September 2018 –
> *The tinnitus started about two weeks ago. Luckily, I can only notice it when I'm in complete silence, so lying in bed etc. However, it does mean that I've finally found a positive to Big G's snoring and incessant grinding of his teeth – once he starts then I can't hear the ringing in my ears!*
> *As for the shingles – for the past four or five days my skin around one side of my midriff has been painful and I had a couple of red patches. As my arms feel bruised on the inside all the time, due to the chemo, I put it down to being more of the same. I had a very fleeting thought about shingles but as I didn't really know much about the virus, I dismissed it as I thought I may be going over the top in finding more things to be wrong with me.*

You really do start to believe that you are conjuring up some of the side effects. Maybe that's another reason for the doctors and nurses not advising you of all the possible side effects…the brain is very influential and I'm sure thoughts can manifest themselves into reality.

5th September 2018 –

Then yesterday, I was watching Dr. Chris on This Morning and he was talking about shingles. He explained that if you've had chicken pox, the virus sits dormant in the nerve tissue near the spinal cord and if your immune system is weakened it might surface as shingles. He said the rash would have little blisters and it is best to get treatment within seventy-two hours.

I thought I should have a look at the red spots, only to find that they had grown into quite a patch, and I also had further patches which spread around my back and into my groin. No wonder I was in pain and finding it difficult to get comfortable! And there were blisters! Off to the doctors I go – and yes, she confirmed it was shingles! I was given a seven-day course of antiviral medication [I ended up having another course for a further seven days], *painkillers to take at night, and instructions to talk to oncology about my next chemo session that I should be having next Monday (10th Sept).*

The next chemo session is when the drugs change and I've been feeling very nervous about it all. Well, I've just had a call back to say they are going to have to delay it for at least a week because of the shingles – and possibly for longer if the blisters haven't scabbed over. Not sure if I am relieved that I don't have to have it on Monday, or fed up that the sick feeling of nervousness will be there for another week!

This morning the rash has spread and is painful, uncomfortable, and looks like a bugger! Sofa and PJs for me today, and possibly no knickers for a week or so due to the blisters in my groin!

Is Karma a bitch? Is someone, somewhere, sticking pins in a doll? If they are, bring it on – you can throw anything you like at me and I will laugh in your face...just as I'm laughing in the face of cancer!

In the end they didn't delay my next session, so I went back to feeling sick and nervous about the new joys that I assumed would come with the new drugs...and boy did they come!

8. Two Weeks on a Roller Coaster. The Ups and Downs of the Cancer Ride!

29th September 2018 –

I seem to have found a bit of a flaw in writing a blog with all the highs and lows of my cancer story – writing about the bad times is not so easy when you are actually going through them – even opening my laptop is too much effort! So, apologies for the radio silence, and worrying some of you (thank you so much for checking up on me), but the last couple of weeks have been a bit of a roller coaster and I just haven't felt like writing, or doing much of anything for that matter. Feeling much more like me again now (not sure that's a good thing – more of me can be too much!)

I think we all retreat into our shells when times are bad, both physically and mentally…and that's ok. We just have to try not to stay there and know that friends and family will accept and love us at our worst…when we don't feel like talking, when we are crying, when we are angry, spiteful or moody…we just need to reach out and accept the help, love, and support.

29th September 2018 –

Monday 10th September – 5th chemo session

Following my blood test on Saturday, I knew there was a question as to whether they would still give me the chemo and I would have to have another blood test before they decided. As this was the first time with the different drugs, the nurses had warned that it would be

Allison was always late for everything. I used to call for her in the morning, in plenty of time, and we always had to rush to high school because she was never ready. Years later, and my poor children had to suffer the consequences – always early for every appointment even though we knew the dentist would be running at least 45-minutes late. One day, when I had dropped Lauren and Kieron at infant school, I was walking out of the gate just as Allison was rushing in with her son…

'You'll make him as paranoid about being late as you made me', was my comment! She is one of the good things to come out of this horror – we'd all but lost touch, apart from on social media, but she reached out to me as soon as she heard and has been a rock, one of many I hasten to add, but that doesn't lessen the love and gratitude I have for her.

Chemotherapy patients have very low immune systems and are very vulnerable to infections and picking up illnesses. This is why I had to be quarantined away from them – the varicella zoster virus, that causes shingles, is contagious.

Not that he has actually tried one, well not that I am aware of! He did, however, look bloody lush in his firefighter uniform which he had kept when he left the service – he obviously knew one day it would be very much appreciated ;)

after 5 o'clock I sat on the sofa, stomach exposed with Big G cleaning the designated area with the antiseptic wipe. He seems calm, although a little hesitant – I, apparently, am not so calm – as at this point, I went into a major meltdown and burst into tears! Not a chance in hell was he coming anywhere near me with that needle! The nurse had told me that if I needed to go to the day unit, at the hospital, to have it done then this would have to be done just before 5pm so I was too late for that. Big G phoned the doctor's surgery to see if anyone could do it there – nope! So, an emergency message went through to one of my ex (hairdressing) clients, and friend, who works at the surgery to see if she was able to come to my rescue, which she did without hesitation – big massive thank you again Jo. Special thanks for making me laugh through the tears by asking me if I wanted the injection in the top, or bottom, roll of fat...charming!

Jo then came round for the next three as well – when you are in a tight spot, people really do step up...so grateful.

29th September 2018 –

My amazing Mum did the last one, and although I was incredibly nervous about a non-professional doing it, she did it without fuss and I wouldn't hesitate letting her do it again, although hopefully it won't be a regular occurrence!

Unfortunately, I had to have them after the next two chemo sessions as well. By the end of it my Mum was a pro. Years ago she had injected my Grandad's insulin when he had stayed with us so she wasn't nervous at all. I'm sure I could do it to someone if I absolutely had to but I was the mother who took her children to Nanna's when they had a plaster that needed ripping off because I couldn't bear the thought of hurting them. I'm also the person who became a hairdresser, not a beautician, because I wouldn't be

31

able to wax or pluck for fear of hurting someone. That will come as a bit of a shock to people as I seem such a bitch on the surface!

29th September 2018 –
A few more tears the same evening [11th September] *as early the next morning Big G was heading off to Zante, for a week, for his niece's wedding. Also, he needed to go and spend some time with Kirstie, his daughter, who was off to Oz for eighteen months. He was really struggling with the idea of leaving me while going through this ordeal but I insisted that he had to go and assured him I would tell him if I needed him to come home at any point (slight lie as you'll see later!), but I knew I would be fine with Lauren and Kieron, and the rest of my family and friends around me...who are all amazing.*

Thursday 13th September –

Mum came with me to see my consultant – a regular appointment, which happens every four weeks.

Although this isn't usually much more than a check in to see how things are going, this time I had a few questions. Warning – men this is about women 'stuff' if you want to skip the rest of this paragraph!! As part of my treatment, I will have hormone therapy to bring on the menopause. This is because the type of breast cancer I have is hormone fed, and only/usually affects pre-menopausal women and this will help prevent it coming back.

I met a lady going through chemotherapy at the same time as me, and for the same type of breast cancer as me, who was post-menopausal. However, I think this is pretty rare.

29th September 2018 –
But the chemo is already affecting my cycle and I've been having a period every other week. For those of you who know me well, you know how much I suffer and so this was one thing I could do without. So, I mentioned this to the consultant and he said we could stop the periods with an injection, Zoladex, every three months – well up for that, now just hoping it works!!

32

It worked like a dream, why hadn't I had this before – a drug that is normally used for treating prostate cancer! I have met a few men since that have this treatment and they actually have menopausal symptoms as well, with hot flushes being the main one – who knew?!

Just thinking back to these appointments…Dr. Ram, my oncology consultant, had not physically examined me. He had looked at scans and mammograms but not once checked my actual boobs…until the day I went in a maxi dress, with a cross over back detail. Every other time I had gone in separates so I could whip my top off, which was quite a habit of mine now, but he didn't want to know. So other than getting practically naked (and showing off my rather attractive nude, anti-chub rub shorts…ladies that don't have a thigh gap will know…) I had to somehow wriggle out of the top part of this dress. Luckily, he left the room at this point. Getting the dress back on was even more comical!

29th September 2018 –

As I only have three chemo sessions left (can't quite believe that), I was curious as to when they would start thinking about surgery. He said they will do another scan and then we could talk about what surgery they are likely to do when I see him next but it will probably happen about four weeks after the last chemo session. All being well, if there are no delays, my last session will be on 12th Nov, which means surgery is likely to be mid-December. Although not ideal, I will just have to get myself organised for Christmas, and then let it all happen around me, which will be a bit tough being as though I'm a 'little' bit of a control freak but pj's and Christmas films sound good recuperation tactics!

The main side effects after the 5th chemotherapy session, apart from feeling generally bleugh and knackered, was a sore, fuzzy mouth and all food tasting disgusting – sort of metally. As you can imagine this slightly took away the enjoyment of the Indian and Chinese we had *for Kieron and Connor's birthday. Although, funnily enough, it hasn't stopped me eating as I am constantly trying to find something that tastes just a little bit nice! Double antibiotics also gave me the runs for over a week...sorry TMI again!*

Although I'd take diarrhoea over constipation any day of the week! To help with the metallic taste, I used plastic baby cutlery. I'm not sure they really helped but anything was worth a go, and they did feel a little better in the fuzzy mouth – not sure how else to describe it!

29th September 2018 –
Monday 17th September –
During chemotherapy, whenever I need to take paracetamol for a headache, I have to take my temperature first. This is in case the headache is an indicator of an infection and taking the paracetamol would bring my temperature down, therefore missing the early signs of infection which can be very dangerous...potentially leading to sepsis. Now I don't always follow this advice but at 2am Monday morning, after feeling (and apparently looking – so Lauren told me at a later date!) very rough all-day Sunday, I woke up with a banging headache and thought I should probably take my temperature. This has to sit between 35.5 and 37.5 degrees Celsius and anything either side of that I have to phone the hospital. So, I took it four times because it was reading 37.6 and 37.7 and then I reluctantly made the call and was told I immediately had to go to A&E. I woke Kieron up, and off we went (via the petrol station - lesson learned hopefully - don't leave your car with less than ten miles of fuel in it when there is a chance of having to do a hospital run in the middle of the night).
Due to the shingles, we were told to sit next to the door away from everyone else. Luckily, we only had to wait about ten minutes before we were called through and I finally ended up in an examination

room where the ambulances bring people in. Firstly, they took bloods...
bottles of blood...not little test tubes...and my god it hurt, to the point
that Kieron told me I was doing well and looked very proud of me!
I mentioned how painful it was to one of the oncology nurses I saw
later in the day and

she said, 'It's because they use knitting needles'! But then I guess
when you are taking so much blood you don't want to use a tiny needle
or you'd be there ages. He then inserted a cannula and I had fluids,
paracetamol and antibiotics (to fight any possible infection as soon
as possible). At 5am, a doctor told me they were keeping me in for at
least twelve hours. This came as a bit of a shock as I was expecting
a shot of antibiotics and to be sent home – I'll expect different if it
happens again! Kieron headed home and at 7.30am I was moved to
an assessment ward which was a hive of activity all day so no sleep for
me, but at least there was plenty to keep me entertained.

During the course of the day, I had a chest X-ray, had to give a
urine sample and they kept talking about me going home soon.

When I went down for the X-ray there was another lady
waiting to go in, and she happened to be the porter's auntie who
had wheeled me, in my bed, to the department. He told me her
story. She had terminal cancer, had even travelled to Spain for
some special treatment but it hadn't worked, and so she was having
palliative treatment. As we left the X-ray area, she told me to 'stay
well'...I instinctively said it back – not much chance of that, she was
dying. This really brought it home that this could have still been my
reality, but she was still wishing me well – what an amazing woman.

29th September 2018 –
Bryony, my sister, works next to the hospital so she had offered
to come and pick me up. As I didn't know what was happening, she
phoned the ward to see how long I would be. Imagine her surprise

when they said they were transferring me to a ward and I was staying in hospital overnight...'Shit' she thought – 'She doesn't know that so now I'm going to have to tell her'! Luckily for Bry, at the same time she was on the phone, the porter, who had taken me to the X-ray, came over and started putting the sides up on my bed and picked my bags up, 'Er, where are we going?'

'To the pub' he said, 'No point as wine tastes disgusting' was my reply – still thinking he was joking about moving me. 'It's not about the taste, it's about the effect,' he said.

'But seriously, where are we going?' – then the nurse arrived to say I had to stay in! That's when the confusion started. The doctor, on the ward we went to, wasn't expecting me and didn't really know why I was there but said I'd definitely be staying in, then he said I might not have to, then I would. To cut a long story short, they eventually set me free at about 7pm and I couldn't run out of there fast enough – well I walked quite slowly as I don't seem to be able to do anything very fast at the moment but you get my gist!

That afternoon I was due to have my first Zoladex injection, to stop my periods and induce the menopause, so I rang the oncology day unit to tell them I was in hospital so wouldn't make my appointment. One of the amazing oncology nurses came over to the ward, at the other end of the hospital, to give it to me so I didn't have to come up another day. She checked with the doctor on the ward that it was OK for me to have it, in case they were going to be administering anything that it would affect, and he said it was fine. After she left, he obviously got a bit confused and came in to double check with me what the injection was for – as the packet said it was for prostate cancer...and I obviously don't even have a prostate! So, I had to explain that I was having it to induce the menopause – see, even as a doctor, every day is a school day (a bit worryingly haha)!

As I was getting ready to leave, a nurse told me not to go anywhere before I had the cannula out – 'er don't worry…funnily enough it makes me feel sick…and where it is in the crook of my elbow means I can't really do anything – so don't panic – I won't take it with me!'

29th September 2018 –
   I didn't tell Big G about my little 'trip' to the hospital, even though I'd promised I would, as I knew I was fine and didn't want him to cut his holiday short – but I was fully prepared to feel the wrath of his anger later – luckily, he was so relieved to be home that he didn't tell me off too much!
   Thursday 20th September –
   On Wednesday I noticed a weird red patch, in the shape of a turtle, on my wrist where my cannula had been for my last chemo – nine days before. As I was going up to the hospital for a scan and mammogram (so the consultants could start thinking about what surgery they would be doing), I called into the day unit for them to have a look at it! Not sure anyone really knew what had caused it other than some sort of delayed reaction to the chemo. They drew around the patch and called for the clinical photographer to take photos of it! Who knew there was such a thing? He said they take photos of anything needed in the hospital, from births to deaths and everything in between, including when someone chopped their hand off with a chainsaw! A doctor also had a look and requested I go back on Monday so she could have another look. By Monday it was a lot redder, a bit sore and itchy, so I had another photo taken and a referral to 'plastics'. I'm not sure why they were referring me there, and stupidly I didn't ask, but I'm hoping they will throw in a free face-lift when I go!

It turned out to be a chemo burn and I got another small one on my hand the next chemo session too. By the time I got an appointment with the plastic surgery team it had healed and they didn't want to mess about with it, and since then it has faded completely.

29th September 2018 –

Then we headed off to the Breast imaging department to have a mammogram first – really not the most pleasant experience, for me or the poor lady who has to get my boob in the right position for it to be squashed to about an inch! Then the scan...last time I had one, the tumour had shrunk to about half the size...this time – NO tumour!! I'm sorry, can I just clarify that...Yes, the tumour has gone!! OMG, that's incredible. I knew this was a possibility, which is why they fitted a clip in the middle of it, before I started chemo, so they would know where to operate, but it was still amazing news – the chemo is working and worth all of the crappiness I feel! This news won't change the 'plan' – I will still have surgery (not sure what yet until I see the consultant again in a couple of weeks), and I will still have the remaining three sessions of chemo, and all the other treatment after the surgery, but it can only mean that things are going in the right direction – up yours, cancer!!

This week has been a good week, as I've felt a lot better and able to catch up with a few people. My next chemo session is on Monday (1st Oct) and I'm hoping not to have any issues this time – haha, very wishful thinking I'm sure but you never know!

9. Aunt Sally – Not the Best Look!

> 11th January 2019 –
>
> *Well, hello there, it's been a while. What a mad few months it has been – so many lows and not too many highs unfortunately. Just wanted to write about the last few sessions of chemo, my surgery, and the next steps...*
>
> *I won't go massively into detail about the last few sessions of chemotherapy (final session 12th Nov), but just wanted to list the new 'surprises' that cropped up in terms of side effects, the little gems...*
>
> *Now I used to love a bit of Worzel Gummidge but looking like Aunt Sally was never on my wish list (OMG I just looked up when it was on TV and it was 1979-1981 – I am sooo old!). But hey, chemo had other ideas and so with the last two sessions I had a week of rosy cheeks. This attractive look was also added to by a red, itchy rash across my chest and neck – oh the joys!*

I guess Aunt Sally was an upgrade from the Uncle Fester look I was mainly modelling up to now – the good looks of Grant Mitchell had long gone by this point!

> 11th January 2019 –
>
> *Another absolute treat was weeping, extremely sore, eyes. Mainly the left one oddly enough and it actually felt red-raw inside. Most nights I took myself to bed by 8pm so that I could try and sleep away a few hours because the pain was pretty unbearable. The first week I put it down to losing my eyelashes, which along with my eyebrows, disappeared with chemo session number six, but the pain continued with the remaining sessions so it was just another perk!*

> *Tip of the week – never leave home without a tissue (or at least a scarf!!) when you don't have any nose hairs. Still slightly annoying though when you have to hold said tissue under your nose whilst unloading your shopping trolley, doing the washing up, putting on socks – dew drips!*

Lauren warned me about the snot as she had plucked all her nose hairs out when she was at uni and had suffered the consequences for weeks after! I'm still a bit paranoid, as I don't think all the hairs have grown back so I'm still inclined to get the odd dew drip. My eyebrows and eyelashes haven't grown back properly either. I did have microblading on the eyebrows but not sure I'll bother again. I'm a bit annoyed that I bought a mascara in anticipation for the regrowth but my eyelashes are about 2mm long, after over three years, so not sure I'm going to be fluttering them any time soon!

> 11th January 2019 –
> *I stayed fairly upbeat through most of the 'chemo journey'. Don't get me wrong I've definitely had a few tears but I think the lack of realisation (still feel like this isn't really happening to me) has saved me from any deep emotions about the whole thing. So, I was totally shocked at the absolute, overwhelming feelings of jealousy that came over me one afternoon...This was after chemo session number six and I was off to Mum's for one of my daily injections. Big G was driving me and as we passed the petrol station, I just felt this wave of emotion and a little bit of 'hate' I guess. The best way to describe it is when you are in the limo going to a funeral of a loved one and you wonder how on earth other people are going about their daily business, happy and smiling, while you are in so much pain. Well, this was me...how on earth could they be filling up their cars, acting normally, when I was 'suffering' so much. This feeling lasted for a couple of days but I then had a very stern word with myself (internally rather than out*

loud – chemo brain is definitely affecting my memory and ability to get words out, but it's not yet sending me bonkers enough that I talk to myself). I know from personal experience that everyone has their own story, their own pain, their own issues and so who am I to judge that they are better off than me, not suffering as much as me. Just because they don't have a forehead that goes from their non-eyelashed eyes right down to their arse crack, does not mean they are all good!

Wow, never a truer statement. Cancer, miscarriage, mental health, anxiety issues, and many other life experiences, have taught me to not judge people. Obviously I'm not a pro at this and still have the odd bitchy moment…lack of understanding…but on the whole I think I am a fairly rounded person who tries to look deeper into why someone may be behaving how they are. For example, I can be larger than life in new, uncomfortable situations; it's either that or sit in the corner and hide; but I'm actually very shy…don't laugh… so I have to put on a show (usually wine induced) to disguise my nerves. In fact, I can be pretty annoying, even unlikeable!

One occasion at a friend's house party, having gone on my own, I drank so much wine that I ended up having detailed conversations with some of the guests about dating and their sex lives! Oh, and that just brought another memory to the forefront – having a 'go' at a restaurant owner in Turkey because he didn't see his kids (couldn't be bothered with the hassle with his ex), having an in-depth conversation, really telling him off – I was really 'going in', and Big G got a tad worried as he'd previously told us about the gun he had behind the bar!

I've learnt over the years to tone it down a bit, thankfully, but the anxiety is massively still there. This has affected me so much that I miss out on social events if I have to go on my own, and then get really cross with myself, knowing that once I was there, I would have had a ball! This is why I really try hard not to judge other people. I get that they may be struggling with whatever is going on in their lives. We all handle the same situations differently. We all deal with our demons in different ways and we all have demons, even if other people can't see them.

Back to the side effects –

11th January 2019 –
Everything was tasting absolutely minging but I was still managing to put on weight – I know...you'd think most people with cancer would lose weight, but actually putting weight on is more common than I realised having looked online (often due to steroids, lack of exercise, and I had the added extra of having a medically induced menopause). I also had excruciating indigestion, a weird taste/smell at the back of my throat, wrinkly fingertips like I'd been soaking in the bath for hours, the stairs looking like Mount Everest when it was time to go up to bed, and other side effects that I took for granted – all in all the last few months of chemo were bloody rubbish. And up to at least four weeks after the last session, I felt lousy, exhausted, and pretty crap continuously really!

Felt, and looked, pretty crap! Looking back at photos I look like a different person – or a monster as I was told after! Lauren didn't usually ask me how I was whenever she came round. One reason was to avoid just talking about cancer all the time, but the main reason was because she could clearly see I wasn't OK so what was the point of banging on about it!

11th January 2019 –
But that bit (chemotherapy) was over...the next hurdle was surgery, which before chemo I thought would be a doddle in comparison but the nearer it got, the more terrified I became!

> *It's very surreal having a conversation with someone as they are looking at, and manhandling, your boobs (reminds me of a visit with a friend to see a surgeon about breast implants, and I found it hilarious watching him talk to her chest, head tipping from side to side)! My surgeon asked if I would be happy to be smaller, as the tumour had been quite large in the bottom half of my right breast – 'yeah that would be great, and if you could put them back in the right place that would be brilliant' was my response!*
>
> *On checking that she had another team of surgeons who could work on my left breast at the same time, I was booked in for a lumpectomy and reconstruction of the right (therapeutic mammoplasty), and reconstruction (reduction mammoplasty) on the left breast so that I wasn't massively lopsided! Well, there has to be a silver lining to having breast cancer – new, smaller, pert boobs were mine! During surgery I would also have sentinel lymph nodes removed (they took two) from my right armpit (the side with cancer) which would be examined, along with all of the breast tissue they removed from both sides.*

Although three years on, not that pert, or small for that matter! And still very lopsided as radiotherapy has shrunk the right one quite a bit!

> 11th January 2019 -
>
> *The morning of the surgery, 6th December 2018, I had blue dye injected into my boob so they could determine which lymph nodes to take. I also had a wire fitted into my boob so the surgeon could see where the centre of the tumour was to ensure they took enough tissue for assessment. By the time I had been drawn on, measured, prodded and poked, the fear of the operation had just about disappeared and I just wanted to get it over with! Big G, on the other hand, looked terrified!!*

While the surgeon was drawing on me, she apologised for having to poke and pull my boobs about. I told her not to worry, and that it must be worse for her. I also had the same conversation with a nurse doing my smear test once – when she apologised, I said it was OK and that it must be worse for her having to poke around in random people's fanwahs! That also reminds me of another smear test when a pubic hair got caught in the spectrum…I tried to tough it out but it hurt so much I had to ask her to release it and start again – the fun us women have to go through! And I never know whether to shave a little, or a lot, before a smear test – I don't want the nurse to think I'm trying too hard! Haha.

But back to the surgeon, she made me laugh telling me about a time when she was a junior doctor and had to use her stethoscope on an elderly lady with massive bosoms. Embarrassed as to how to get to her heart, the patient took her boob and put it over her shoulder. Half way through the examination the boob fell down, trapping the stethoscope – completely embarrassing the doctor. 'Don't worry', said the lady and promptly flung it back over her shoulder! Clearly you had to be there – not so funny writing it down – but the story certainly helped to ease the tension!

The other amusement from that day came from the porter taking me on a magical mystery tour around the hospital – it was his first day and after the dye and wire was fitted, I wasn't allowed to walk, so I was to be wheeled back to the ward before surgery. But he took me to the wrong ward, at the other end of the hospital, and me and Big G were too polite to question him, even though we were pretty sure he was going the wrong way!

11th January 2019 –
    After surgery, when I woke up in the recovery room, I was surprised to recognise an old friend. He didn't, however, recognise me (he actually checked the computer records to check it was really me!!) and it wasn't until he wheeled me into the lift (surrounded by mirrors) on the way

> *to the ward that I could see why – not sure I was looking my best at this point and it had been a few years since I had last seen him – no hair, no eyebrows, no lenses or make-up, and a few extra wrinkles and pounds, is not the best version of me!! I had to stay in hospital for one night because my wounds had leaked quite a bit, as they continued to do for another few days. When I got changed into my pyjamas that night, I looked down and said to Big G that I was really swollen after the surgery – imagine my horror when I realised that wasn't the case. What I could actually see was my rolls of fat that had previously been hidden by my big, droopy, boobs!*

Two days after my surgery Lauren had a Christmas party at her flat and I was determined to attend. Gingerly, I managed the two flights of stairs and got stuck into the sex on the beach – our go-to cocktail. In hindsight, mixing alcohol and painkillers may not have been the best idea but I had the best evening, forgot my troubles for a few hours, and even became a polar bear whilst playing Charades! When I got home and undressed there was blood everywhere…mmm maybe crouching down to be a polar bear hadn't helped – I didn't admit this to the nurse when she changed my dressing after they suggested I go straight to the hospital, even though it was the middle of the night. Luckily all was ok, and my stitches were still in place!

> *11th January 2019 –*
> *So having already been for a few dressing changes, I went for an appointment at the breast clinic for them to check me over. The check-up was done by one of the surgeons who had operated on me and he wanted to know which boob had leaked most – clearly wanting to know who was the better stitcher-upper...not competitive at all!!! Haha. He then said to the nurse, who was going to change my dressings, 'Can you check that the nipples are still alive' (they*

> are removed and sewn back in the right place but they can die and
> fall off!).
>
>   'OMG you really need to rephrase that – that is disgusting' was my
> response – luckily, he laughed and said he'd work on his terminology!!
> When I mentioned it to one of the oncology nurses later that day she
> said 'Well at least if you stand on something strange, you'll know what
> it is'!

In such terrifying, upsetting and unknown circumstances, inappropriate humour from the team around me (family, friends, consultants, surgeons, nurses and all the NHS and supporting staff) really got me through. And when I say they are 'sewn back in the right place', my nipples are different sizes, different shapes, and point in different directions. Not that I'm complaining, much! But at least they 'survived' – a lot don't. Funnily enough they still react to touch and cold (not so handy) even though they are numb and I have no feeling in them!

> 11th January 2019 –
>   Five weeks after surgery I am still sore but definitely improving.
> I can just about sleep on my side, with the aid of pillows, but still have
> another three weeks of wearing a bra night-and-day which is not
> normal for me – I am someone who takes my bra off the minute I walk
> in the house! [Mmm, maybe that's why I didn't end up with pert
> boobs! The minute I could go braless, I did! And I still have pain in
> my right boob due to the radiotherapy, three years on.]
>   On the 21st Dec I had my follow up appointment to go through
> the next steps of treatment and to get the results of the analysis they
> had done on the tissue and lymph nodes – I was told that there was
> no cancer and the chemo had got rid of it even before the surgery....
> Best Christmas present EVER! But now neither I, nor the family, can
> play the cancer card – sorry Lauren!! Haha.

Just to reassure you – we did actually continue to play the cancer card fully as my work colleagues will confirm! Well for goodness' sake, if you can't play on having a life-threatening illness, what good is it to anyone – at least something useful had to come from it! And now I can, unfortunately, play too many other cards as well!

11th January 2019 –
What next...well on Wed 16th January 2019 I start three weeks of radiotherapy (fifteen sessions), which is every day (Mon-Fri). I will have another twelve Herceptin injections (one every three weeks), Zoladex injections (one every three months) for the next two years to halt my periods, and hormone tablets every day (along with Calcium and Vitamin D supplements as the hormone tablets can cause osteoporosis [unfortunately a bone density scan shows they have anyway so another pill (Alendronic Acid) for that, for which I oddly have to stand up for half an hour after taking!]) *for the next ten years! But all these treatments are preventative – to hopefully stop the cancer coming back.*

So now it's the New Year and things are looking so much better – still a long way to go and I know there will be many challenges along the way but I am very positive for the future. Emotions took over on NYE and I burst into tears in the middle of Auld Lang Syne, which set Big G off, but I think it must have just been the overwhelming relief that the worst was behind me! And my hair is growing back – in the areas I'd rather it didn't as well unfortunately!! And now I just need to build up some stamina – this time next year...

A bit of a list of my side-effects – I'm sure it's not exhaustive as I know I've forgotten (deliberately) some of them:

Heartburn – Omeprazole to the rescue...I was literally trying to cave my chest in to stop the pain; Hair fell out; Head hurt when my hair started to fall out, and when it rained...ouch; Constipation; Diarrhoea; Incontinence; Weird smell/taste at back of throat; Sore eyes; Feeling faint; Extreme fatigue; Wrinkly fingertips; Being (luckily only once) and feeling sick; Sweaty; and head/body that felt like a dead weight when I woke up – you know when you fall asleep on your arm and it goes dead…well that's how my whole body and head felt most mornings, very odd.

Also, Chemo burns; Shingles; Bird poo stain on my scalp!; Aunt Sally cheeks; Rashes; Ulcers and sore mouth; Very dry skin; Forearms felt bruised inside; Joints hurt like an old lady's body – I actually get jealous when I see someone crouch down and get up without having to crawl to something to push themselves up on, still!

I also had a low immune system; had to crawl up the stairs sometimes, everyday tasks became a real challenge; Metallic taste; Fuzzy mouth; Dry mouth; Nails weakened due to chemo and reaction to light (so I had a manicure and gel nails every three weeks as suggested by the doctors, bonus); Needed to keep out of the sun due to chemo and radiotherapy; Running nose, constantly; Weight gain and swollen body; burnt boob (radiotherapy, pain and skin peeling); Generally looked and felt like shite!

10. To Ring or Not to Ring?

6th February 2019 –

Yesterday was my last radiotherapy. Three weeks of going up to Ipswich hospital every day apart from Saturdays and Sundays. But yet again, the staff made it as comfortable and 'fun' as it could possibly be – I really can't praise them enough.

The first step of treatment is a 'planning scan' where they work out the area that needs zapping. During this appointment I was given three tattoos – unfortunately not pretty flowers or butterflies – just three black dots so the machine could be lined up perfectly. Then two weeks later I went for my first treatment...

Everyone says radiotherapy is a doddle after chemotherapy so I wasn't too worried about it. Getting on the bed and into position was not the easiest or the most dignified – arms raised above my head on the red arm-rests, bum behind a metal plate, and knees over the blue rest thingy (technical term I'm sure). I had my own special and very attractive gown that I took home and brought back to wear each day, which enabled my boob to be popped out easily, along with all the tattoos. I was slightly embarrassed about the underarm hair that has now come back (why couldn't chemo have killed those follicles permanently??!!). They had told me not to wet-shave before having radiotherapy and I do not have an electric razor – however, I rectified that after the first session by pinching Big G's – well if he didn't know before, he knows now!!

Then the radiologists started pulling and pushing me, lining up the tattoos, randomly saying numbers to each other, getting me in the correct position. My appointments were all early in the morning, so I had the disadvantage of them having very cold hands most of the time! And what is it about being told you can't move and getting the worst itch on your nose, or on the back of your neck, just like when

Since treatment I have to be very careful in the sun – chemotherapy and radiotherapy thins the skin, so factor 35 or 50 it is. The first day I was in Crete with Bryony, about two months after I'd finished radiotherapy, I just sprayed suntan lotion on the skin on show, as you would, only to realise that my right boob was tanning through my costume/boobtube. So now I have to make sure I spray before I get dressed!

There is a bell in the radiotherapy department that someone donated for patients to ring to signify the end of treatment (like I'm sure you've seen on the advert about childhood cancers). When I was having chemo I heard it rung a few times and it made me smile. Now you would think it would be something I would rush to do; however, something was holding me back. One reason being that I'm not really at the end of my treatment – I've still got Herceptin injections every three weeks, Zoladex injections every three months, heart scans, and Hormone therapy for ten years – So was it right for me to ring it? But the main thing that worried me about ringing it was being very conscious that other people were still having their treatment and that they may not get the all clear at the end of it. When I finished chemo I left the clinic very quietly, as I knew some people were there to help prolong life rather than for a cure, and so I felt very uneasy about celebrating too loudly that I was through that bit.

There was a lady who had the same appointment time for chemo for quite a few of my sessions. She was there for palliative care and she told me the only reason she was still having treatment was due to family pressure, and her daughter wanting her Mum to see her graduate the following summer – she had wanted to stop the treatment a while ago because it made her feel so ill. Now I totally get this, and I'm sure I used to feel the same before my diagnosis, but surely the person with cancer (or other life-limiting illness) should be able to decide about their own treatment without added pressure? I get the pressure from loved ones if there is every chance you will survive with treatment, and I would have walked to the moon and back, over hot coals (it felt like I did at times), to take every bit of treatment they threw at me…but if you know you are dying from it, you are exhausted, you are in pain, surely you should decide?

6th February 2019 –

And I was feeling very much the same about the bell yesterday. But the receptionist thought I should ring it, the radiologists thought I should ring it, Bryony wanted a photo of me ringing it, and I thought I may regret it if I didn't! So, although I was feeling very conflicted, I gave it one, very quiet and very quick, 'ding' and felt very silly, and left as soon as I could.

But that's another thing ticked off the list...and I'm doing ok! I'm a bit worried that others will expect me to be back to normal fairly soon, and I hope to God I am, but I know this is a very long process. The Zoladex injections are forcing me into the menopause so the hot flushes (power surges) are coming thick and fast. I'm not sleeping at all well due to these (sweaty Betty), pain from the 'sunburn' and still quite a bit of discomfort from the operation, along with the hormone therapy that is starting to make my joints hurt like hell, so also not ideal...

11.   Back to 'Normal'?

4th March 2019 –
'How are you?'
'I'm good thank you'
'So it's all gone? You are all better, back to normal now?'
'Yep, I'm all good'

Well that is a big fat lie – 'normal'...I literally have no idea what normal is now! But what else could I have said?

Maybe...

'No, nowhere near better and nowhere near normal. Yes, the cancer has gone (and trust me I am soooooo happy and grateful for that) but...

- *I'm still in a lot of pain from the operation*
- *I'm still in a lot of pain from the radiotherapy* [and that doesn't really go – still in pain three years on]
- *My body does not look like mine. I may have 'better' boobs, but they are scarred and I have different shaped nipples that point in different directions. I've also got scars from the chemo burns, the shingles and the lymph node clearance*
- *I still have to go for injections – one every three weeks, and another sort every three months*
- *Because of one of the injections, I have to go for heart scans every three months which entails two injections of radioactive stuff into my veins, as although the Herceptin is helping to prevent the cancer coming back, it may severely affect the function of my heart*

- *I have to be careful not to develop lymphedema which is a lifelong, painful, and debilitating condition – so no blood pressure tests, blood tests, injections in my right arm (the side where the lymph nodes were removed), and I also have to be very wary of bites, scratches and any sort of injury to that arm*
- *Most of the time I can hardly move, and I look like I'm ninety-seven, because my joints hurt so much due the hormone treatment, which I have to take for ten years*
- *Along with the pain, the hot flushes brought on by the medically induced menopause mean that I am hardly sleeping*
- *Exhaustion hits me like a bus sometimes and although I want to be able to do everything I did before, I know I can't*
- *My hair may be growing back but it doesn't stop people staring. I feel like holding up a sign to say that I've had cancer, I really don't think I'm young and edgy with this style!*
- *Chemo brain is still affecting me – I can't find the words I'm looking for, I find it difficult to make sense of certain things, I'm very forgetful. And yes, I was like that a bit before, as most of us are, but nothing quite like this!*
- *Although I can now go on holiday, I have to avoid the sun and am limited where I can go due to still having a low immune system (not to mention the fact that flipping travel insurance is higher!)*
- *I'm trying to live without the constant fear that the cancer may come back. I can't live in blissful ignorance anymore that it won't happen to me – it bloody has, and may again [and I know that other things can still happen to me, and my loved ones!]*

...so no, I'm not really back to normal yet – and to be honest, I'm not sure if I ever will be'.

Not sure that is the answer anyone would want to hear so 'Yep, I'm all good' is the response I will continue to give. But then I didn't understand about all of the after effects of cancer treatment either.

I also assumed that once chemotherapy, surgery, and radiotherapy were over, then you would be back to 'normal' however slow that process may take.

That all being said, 'normal' is a funny idea – do I actually want to be back to normal. Surely, I should want to live each day like it's my last because I can really vouch for the fact that we don't know what is around the corner. But then that's not normal life, so should I want to go back to worrying about the simple things like cleaning the house, what to have for dinner etc.? But then if I don't make the most of every second, am I throwing away the good fortune of getting shot of this bastard disease? I guess I have to find a happy medium – anyone got any suggestions how you do that?

So many buts...and what ifs...if we could see into the future, would we want to? Many people have commented on my positivity throughout this ordeal. I'm not sure about positivity, but I've tried to find the humour in each situation, looked on the bright side, made a joke about everything – but in all honesty it's been the only way I could handle it. But there have been moments when I've not managed this...

Last week I sent Big G a text:
'What do I do if the cancer comes back?'
'It won't', he replied.
'You don't know that'
'But they do' (the doctors – well they don't actually!)
'But what do I do if I just get cancer again then?'
I'm not sure he knew how to answer, there was no right answer. Trying to placate me and tell me everything would be fine was not what I wanted, nor would it have been the truth because we simply don't know that. I realise he, and everyone else who loves me, also has to learn to live with the fear.

To be honest, I'm not living with it, the fear, all the time as part of me has gone back to 'blissful ignorance' that it won't happen to me – but part of me has it in the back of my mind constantly. I knew these feelings were likely to come as other people, who have been *through it, have told me that it is after you've finished treatment that somehow the whole thing seems harder – who knew?! During active treatment, the cancer was all consuming with trips to the hospital, side effects of the treatment, medication...but now the hospital visits are less frequent (although I feel 'lucky' that I still have contact with the oncology team because of the injections) and I am starting to go back to work, and therefore, somehow, have to adapt to this new normal.*

I feel this has been a 'moany' blog post, sorry – not much humour in it I'm afraid! But I also feel it's important to share the bad with the good because how do we know

about the aftermath if no one talks about it?

Please believe that I am very happy to be on the right side of this 'story' and I plan to stay well, and I am also excited to be able to start getting back to real life. But I'm a bit worried that people will expect me to be completely 'Mel' again...I'll get there, just bear with me!

What is 'normal' anyway? Everyone's normal has been affected over the last couple of years (Covid-19 2020–22). Some have thrived, some have suffered massively – who knows how you will handle any situation? One day at a time? Reading and digesting every bit of information available? Showing your vulnerable side? Being 'strong'? Wanting to be on your own? Needing people around you? There is no right or wrong way – there is just your way, and that's OK!

12. Just Ow!

15th March 2019 –

Last Friday, I had a MUGA heart scan to check if the Herceptin injections (given every three weeks to help prevent the cancer reoccurring) are having any negative effects on my heart function.

I was feeling very nervous about the process, although I have had it done twice before. I was probably even more nervous, if anything, as chemo progressively impacts negatively on the veins. You would think I would be used to needles by now but it never gets easier. And because I had some lymph nodes removed on my right side, they can only use the veins in my left arm – and they had to find two!

I'm all 'brave' going in for the first injection of radioactive stuff, chatting ten to the dozen...slight verbal diarrhoea! After the normal questions, ID check [this made me laugh on every appointment – like I'd put myself through this if I didn't have to!] and signing to say I'm not pregnant (haha!) etc., she starts looking for a vein in the normal places, being the back of the hand and crook of the elbow. Nope, nothing usable there! So, she then decides to go in on the inside of my forearm. Yuck and bloody OW, that flipping hurts!

'Oh, I've failed. I'll have to try again'.

At this point my voice wobbled and then, from nowhere, I burst into floods of tears – cried like a baby! The nurse was so lovely, apologising for not getting in the vein, and I'm apologising for crying, with us both laughing at the situation.

She said, 'I'd better not hug you because apparently I'm really good at hugs, so it will make you cry more'.

At this point another nurse came in, I think she wondered what on earth she had come in to! Once I had calmed down, she had to try again and the only place she could find a vein was the inside of my wrist – OMG double yuk and double OW! But success and now just a *half hour wait before going through it again before the scan. Luckily the next one went straight in the vein, no issues but quite a bit of OW!*

Then in the afternoon, I had the pleasure of my Zoladex implant being injected into my stomach. Big G is fabulous and will always joke to try and relieve my worries, but even he was shocked about the size of the needle – so another flipping OW!

But at least I have three months before having to do either of these again...Or so I thought!

I was due to go for my Herceptin injection this afternoon but got a phone call yesterday evening to say they need to cancel it due to the MUGA heart scan showing reduced function. Normal left ventricular ejection fraction (LVEF) is 55% – 70%, and mine has gone down from 66% to 43%! LVEF of 40% or less is classed as heart failure so obviously they have to suspend my treatment. I now have to go for another heart scan (oh deep joy) in about six weeks to assess whether the function has improved so we can continue with the treatment – bit gutted as this will probably mean more regular scans, instead of them being three monthly, and the three treatments that have been postponed so far will have to be added on to the end, so I won't finish the treatment when I thought I would. But hey, hopefully my heart function will get back to normal levels soon and as always, I'm eternally grateful for the care and treatment I am getting from our wonderful NHS.

The break did the trick and then it was all systems go for the rest of the Herceptin injections. They did affect my heart function again but this was discovered at Addenbrooke's hospital much later (and another story) and so it did not halt the treatment again – and finally now I can say it genuinely is all back to normal, or at least it was the last time I was checked!!

13. Stop the Merry-Go-Round, I Want to Get Off

8th May 2019

The past few weeks have definitely felt like a theme park ride, with many highs and a few lows, and sometimes (well most of the time) I'm very bored with the ride and I just want to get off!

Before starting back at work, I wanted to fit in a couple of trips away... I've missed my holidays soooo much. The first trip was Big G and me returning to our piece of paradise, our cave house in Spain [cave house I hear you say – keep reading and I'll tell you more]. I was very worried about what state we were going to find it in, as we've not been since last April [2018] and we left the windows open for ventilation – thinking we would return a few months later. Luckily it wasn't too bad – the fly screens had stopped most of the dust going in. We had such a relaxing time, lots of vino tinto and tapas, sitting by the log burner, looking at 'my' mountains, and time with friends, a proper charge up of my batteries.

Then my sister, Bryony, and I went to Crete for ten days. Brrr, it was a bit chillier than expected so I had to sit in the sun to keep warm! I'm not really meant to sit in the sun after my chemo but Vitamin D is good for you, as I kept telling myself, and I was very sensible about applying the sun cream regularly. I was very pleased with how much walking I managed on the few days we went out, but painful joints (due to the hormone treatment) meant I had to take it easy when I could. At one point Bryony had me climbing over a wall, which would have made 'video of the week' on 'You've Been Framed', but I drew the line at walking down 50 steps just to have my photo taken (which I knew I would hate), knowing I'd have to walk straight back up them! After all, who wants to see photos of themselves as an almost 49-year-old, bald, fat 'bloke' – better to imagine that I am a svelte 30-year-old, with long flowing locks – it's clearly the photos and mirrors that lie! We laughed so much throughout our stay; we will have to make it a yearly jaunt!

Bloody Covid-19 got in the way of this…maybe next year!

8th May 2019 –

The day after we got back, I had to go for my heart scan to check if the heart function had gone up so I could resume the Herceptin injections. After the last time I was incredibly anxious, but I popped an anti-anxiety pill that the hospital gave me, and luckily, they had no problems finding the veins this time. And good news, I heard today that it is back up to fifty-five, so I can start the injections again next week – mmm something to look forward to!

I had already been back into work, for a morning or so, a week before I went on holiday, but Monday 29th April was the first day I was going back in properly since starting treatment – to do actual work, albeit for only two mornings a week to start with. Bearing in mind that it has almost been a year since I was there, this was a pretty momentous day. My emotions were all over the place – anxiety, pride, fear, and happiness. The journey there involved quite a few tears, then lots of hugs and smiling faces from colleagues which was amazing (thank you so much guys), telling me how good I looked - slap on, drawn on eyebrows, big earrings, fake it till you make it! Then, seemingly from nowhere a total engulfing feeling of being overwhelmed whilst sitting at my desk – what the chuff am I doing back, I can't even remember my own name sometimes, let alone function well in my job! Luckily, there was just my manager and me in the office at the time, and she was fab, as she has been all the way through this (thanks Josie), so I let myself cry and then got on with the morning!! I think the anxiety will continue for a while, but I felt better when I went back in, and I'm sure it will get easier. There were a few jokes about playing the 'cancer card' at work, especially when I was being 'bullied' into holding a mouse and a gerbil (er no thanks, minging creepy tails) and tried to get out of it. Although I should have been more careful re the risk of lymphedema but hey, I forgot - well surely, it's a good thing that cancer isn't on my mind constantly (although I guess it should be a little more at times!). [For a bit of context here, I worked in a college at the time which had an Animal Care course, and there were lots of different animals about!!]

The next day I started the 'HOPE' course, which is run by Macmillan, and helps you cope with life after a cancer diagnosis. I've not used their facilities or services at all throughout, but have been having moments of panic about the future etc. so thought why not give it a go. I fully expected to hate it and not go after the first week – I still don't want cancer buddies – but actually it was really nice to know I'm not the only one feeling this way, emotionally and physically. When I arrived, early of course, I felt a bit sick sitting in the car park. I get social anxiety in new situations (I'm very good at hiding it) but as soon as a car pulled up next to me, I had to laugh – there was a lady with hardly any hair, well she's clearly going to the same place as me!!

The Cancer Club (as we renamed the group) ladies are amazing. Throughout the course we joked (inappropriately of course), laughed, cried, and supported each other. We have a WhatsApp group and still now meet up for coffee/lunch occasionally. It is so freeing to be able to be honest and moan about our feelings, fears, and anxieties, without feeling guilty and worrying the family, and to have other people that can actually relate to our thoughts and feelings.

8th May 2019 –
Thursday, in the same week, was a mixed day! Joy at spending time with our new great niece, frustration at driving around Cambridge to look at new cars with Big G, his sister and his dad (confusion all around), excited to be feeling well and almost energetic – I should have stopped at that and known that it had been a long day! But oh no, I thought I was all good, and as Big G was off to visit his daughter in Australia, and Thursday evening would be our only opportunity to go out before he went, I decided it would be a good idea to go out for a meal and a few wines! All was well until I had finished my meal – G was still going (haha), well it was a buffet – and a wave of tiredness hit like a bus.

> 'We are going to have to go. I can't be here anymore', then the tears started!
>
> Not embarrassing at all in a restaurant, I felt a right tit (got to love a good pun!). The tears were clearly aided and abetted by the red wine, but I felt so upset, so desperate, that I couldn't even last an evening without feeling so tired, so ill, so not 'me'. More tears followed at home, when the hell am I going to be 'back to normal', when the hell can I do more than one thing a day without feeling shite. I absolutely know it is a matter of time and the importance of being kind to myself in the meantime. I also know that I will never fully be the old me, and that's ok. But at times it really gets to me, and I also know that's ok because the next day will be better – well actually the day after this was spent in bed – but the day after was better!

Fatigue and tiredness still do hit me like a bus sometimes but this is only occasionally – thank goodness.

> 8th May 2019 –
>
> I have to keep reminding myself that my body, and mind, are amazing – they have got me through this last year and as one of the ladies at the HOPE course said 'We are rock stars' – and I know patience is the key, one step at a time, just setting realistic goals, appreciating what I have, where I'm at, how much I've been through and that I am coming out the other side.

14. Does Everything Really Happen for a Reason?

Life has many twists and turns. If you are like me, you try to find reasons and justifications for the shite stuff – weird how we usually just accept the good stuff!

24th August 2016 –

> We are all fantastic; please don't let the daily grind make you forget that.
>
> There are many sayings and phrases that we use on a daily basis, that help us understand or justify ours, and other people's actions, and how we view the world. Do you consider yourself as a glass half empty or glass half full kind of person?
>
> I was watching 'Made in Chelsea' with Lauren this morning and one of the guys said something that made us both laugh, and then it got me thinking. He was referring to his hair receding and it went something like 'The way I look at it...I'm not losing hair; I am gaining face' – talk about looking on the bright side! So, I started wondering what sort of person I am, half full...or half empty kind of gal? And what other sayings relate to how we live our lives?
>
> Most of the time I would say I look at life with a glass half full outlook. I don't really see the point in looking for the negatives and dwelling on the bad stuff. But that isn't to say that I can maintain this all of the time, and I definitely haven't at certain times of my life.

And I definitely don't at night-time! I can't rationalise what day of the week it is at 3am so I tend to think the worst about all situations when I should be fast asleep!

24th August 2016 –

We all have 'duvet' days, or even weeks, where we struggle to get off the sofa, struggle to see anything positive in the circumstances we find ourselves in, and the glass certainly appears half empty. And I think that's OK, it really is all right to allow yourself to have these times and 'wallow' for a while, but not for too long (I am in no way referring to depression when I say this, which is completely different). At some point you have to pick yourself up, jump in the shower, put your face on and get back to real life – and although this may feel forced the first time or two, hopefully the front you put on will become natural and the glass will begin to appear half full again.

'Fake it till you make it' became my motto during, and since, my cancer diagnosis. I, sometimes, felt pressure (more from myself than those around me) to 'perform', be better, look to the future, and so faking it was the way I handled it and eventually it started to become my reality again.

24th August 2016 –

I do try to live believing 'everything happens for a reason' and definitely consider that this is true in the majority of cases. Like if you don't get the dream job, the dream house, even the dream boyfriend – it just means the next one that comes along will be so much better and you will look back and be so chuffed that you didn't get 'it'! This has happened to me on more occasions than I could mention (clearly, I am talking about jobs and houses...I've never had to beat the 'boys' away with a stick!). But how can this still be true when you are talking about natural disasters, accidents, or people dying from illness? How can you possibly find the reason for these? So maybe the saying is only relevant for the small things that happen in our lives...the things that we think matter but in the grand scheme of things really don't! Maybe another phrase is more appropriate – don't sweat the small stuff?

> *You learn something new every day. Life is a lesson and every single day something new happens; so, open your eyes, your mind, and your heart. It allows you to truly experience every new sensation with enthusiasm and interest. Easier said than done I know, but just try to remember, especially when the going gets tough (the tough get going... sorry, can't say/type that without wanting to burst into song!), that you woke up this morning when far too many people didn't. I firmly believe than when someone dies before their time it HAS to be a reminder to the rest of us to live our lives to the fullest. It may sound like a selfish thing to say but I am sure that these people would say the same if they could come back for ten minutes. Life really is for living, and life really is way too short...so read a book, go for a walk, pick a buttercup, appreciate the small stuff, and tell those around you that you love them.*

It's funny reading this back since having my cancer diagnosis. I'm not sure if I really believed the words that I wrote...life is for living, live each day like it's your last – blah blah blah. Did I really live like that, or did I still worry about whether the ironing was done, whether the house was clean, whether I was a size 10 (haha never worried enough to do much about it apart from when I was getting married to Big G)? I have to admit that I could talk the talk, but definitely didn't walk the walk – no, we'd better not go on holiday; no, we'd better not buy new sofas; no, we'd better not go out for a slap-up meal. Mostly the reason was lack of money, or my perception of lack of money. Don't get me wrong, there were many times when I didn't have a bean to my name and had to hide from the milkman (even the kids remember the fun and games of those times), but there were definitely times that I put the kibosh on things when I could have just 'lived a little' and said 'sod it'!

Even since my diagnosis I've been waiting for the moment when I say 'sod it, let's go for it – let's backpack round the world and just see what happens.' It's been over four years and I'm only just getting there – not sure about the backpacking (although we've already bought a couple of backpacks so we are going to have to at some point…mmm, maybe that was a 'sod it' moment – thought about the backpacks and two days later they arrived in post) – but I have given up work, sold the house, and bought a campervan, so I guess it's only a matter of time before we jet/drive off – get going, doing, living!

Just a thought…when do we stop really living like each day is special? As kids, we don't have all the worries that come with adulthood (I know childhood comes with its own worries/anxieties, especially these days), and we just crack on. A memory of mine is leaving my house at about 6am (I was under seven) to walk over to my friend's house across the road so I could jump on her mum and dad's bed. Problem was she didn't answer the door so I had to go home. You can imagine my mum's horror when she answered the front door to me barefoot and in my nightie, probably only five minutes later! She thought I'd been sleep walking so I had to tell her what I'd been up to – I think she wanted to cry with relief that she didn't have to start bolting the doors to keep me in at night.

24th August 2016 –
Life is like an echo, what you send out comes back (karma I guess) – so be nice! Do good things, use kind words, but not just to get good things back from others. When you are nice it gives you positive feelings anyway – getting a 'thank you' or a smile from family, a friend, a partner, a stranger, is an amazing sensation. It doesn't cost anything but the rewards are priceless – so give that compliment, go that extra mile, make someone's day just a little better by having you in it.

The best way to have the life you want is to want the life you have – how true is this? Same idea as the 'grass is not greener' I guess. Of course, it is always a good thing to strive for better things, a better life, a better future, but only up to a point. There is nothing wrong with wanting the best for you and your family but we should all take the time to look around us and appreciate what we already have. Other people may appear to have more, be happier, thinner, taller, prettier... but let me assure you that someone looks your way and thinks all of those things, and more, about you (maybe not the thinner/prettier in my case). So, quash the jealousy, it is neither attractive nor healthy – be happy for others, but much more importantly, be happy for you and yours – I am!

Life will always throw us challenges and we never know how strong we can be until we don't have any other choice – oh so flipping true!

15. Mum – Seriously, Who Did Know What Would Happen?

A blog post written by Lauren

1st July 2019 –

The day that mum got diagnosed, I knew something was wrong as soon as I saw her. She wasn't crying. She didn't look visibly upset. She didn't say anything. And up until this point she had kept her mum-head firmly on, never hinting that anything could be wrong beforehand in the hope to save us from unnecessary worry. But that day I just knew. I knew that something wasn't right, and I knew that whatever it was, it wasn't small.

Not only is mum the person I know the most in the world; she's also the person that's most like me in the world, and so whilst it's difficult trying to explain how I knew, it really just came down to knowing her habits and mannerisms so well, that I knew she was acting strange within a split second of seeing her. Because her habits and mannerisms are my habits and mannerisms.

When I still lived at home and used to get home from work, I always had the same routine. I hate to sound so predictable, but as a creature of habit and a seeker of cosiness, these same five steps happened every single day:

I would stick my head in the lounge and quickly say 'Hi' to let whoever was in there know that I was home.

I would walk into the dining room to throw my shoes and bag down in a random spot (which wasn't where they ever belonged, but I continued to do it anyway).

My bra would then immediately come off and PJs would go on.

The kettle would be switched on. Snacks would be sourced.

I'd then go back into the lounge (often joining Mum), bust out a blanket, and put the recliners up.

And these weren't just my five steps. These were Mum's five steps as well. My routine didn't deviate; her routine didn't deviate. Finding Mum in any other way than in the step-five-position would have been weird that evening, because one of the many things that we have in common is that we like to be comfy. We often joke about how horrendously crap and lazy we'll be in retirement and how we'll never be those well put-together people who do their hair, makeup, and get dressed perfectly every day without fail, no matter if they have any plans or not; just like my lovely Nanna (Mum's mum) does.

Nanna is never found slouching. Nanna is never found super casual. Nanna is always ready for anyone to pop round unexpectedly without the last-minute panic of wiping smudged mascara off her face. Nanna is who we aim to be like in retirement but know that we will never actually be like because we can't even manage it now.

And whilst it may seem like I've gone off topic a bit and you're probably wondering why I'm talking about my Nanna, I haven't at all. Because Nanna was the reason that I knew.

The routine that day got shortened from the usual five steps, to this:

I would stick my head in the lounge and quickly say ~~'Hi' to let whoever was in there know that I was home.~~ 'Why are you being weird? You're sat like Nanna'.

That's it. There were no other steps.

Everything stopped.

The world stopped.

And it really did.

We were confused. We were shocked. We were scared.

But then, the world started spinning again.

The world started to pick up the pace.

Life began to happen again.

Because Mum might have had cancer, but she wasn't dead. She was well and truly alive, and so we were sure as hell not going to allow her entire world to become about cancer and cancer alone.

I know many of the people reading this won't know me in person, or if you do, maybe not that well. Instead, many of you will be old friends of Mums, or people she has met or spoken to within the past year since this all began. Therefore, here's a bit of background about me:

I'm not exactly the best at managing my emotions and anxieties (those that do know me personally are currently laughing their arses off at how much of an understatement that statement actually is, I'm sure).

Let's put it this way: When psychologists say that we have both 'Fight or Flight' responses to situations, I've always wondered whether or not I was actually built with the ability to 'fight', as when afraid, I always magically grow the most large and powerful wings you could ever imagine, and they get me the fuck out of whatever situation I'm in as quickly as humanly possible. I panic. I avoid. I run.

It's my default. It's my coping mechanism. It's often my worst enemy.

But through this, my brain and my ability to hide from the truth has been my best friend. We made jokes, we learnt not to talk about cancer every single day, and we kept things normal. We talked about insignificant things. She asked me about my friends. We spoke about the family. We talked about anything that wasn't cancer. Except for occasionally (and when I say occasionally, I mean regularly) playing the cancer card, because why wouldn't you?

I rarely asked her how she was or if she was OK.

I could see how she was, she looked like shit. I knew she would tell me if she was really struggling and needed anything, and so I knew that I didn't need to ask. Just the initial few days of talking about cancer was draining, and we knew we couldn't continue like that long term, for any of our sakes.

Everyone else was nice enough to ask mum daily how she was, and whilst appreciated, I felt like she deserved at least one person that was acting like nothing had changed. At least one person that wouldn't be afraid to take the piss when she struggled to get up from the sofa. At least one person who wouldn't treat her like she was going to break. And at least one person that would compare her to a Mitchell brother, which she undoubtedly did look like, but no one else would have the audacity to say it.

It's not kicking a woman when she's down, it's jokingly kicking a woman all the time and not stopping when she's down. That's our relationship. That's our humour. So, it was about still having a laugh, still being cheeky, and still treating her like my mum, because she still was my mum. Even in the worst of it all. Even when her body looked as though it was going to fail her. And she gives as good as she gets, by the way.

In terms of letting it sink in for myself though, there were really only four times where I was properly scared or fully admitted that Mum even had cancer. The rest of the time I was in complete denial.

I felt the cancer the day after she got diagnosed. I got out of bed at 7am and rushed to the shops to buy every cancer-fighting food I could find in the hope that I could cure her instantly.

I felt the cancer around a week after she was diagnosed when Jess Glynne's song 'I'll Be There' made it number 1 into the charts – honestly, listen to that song whilst thinking of cancer and it will absolutely destroy you. Apologies in advance.

I felt the cancer when I was ready to move out and I had this illogical meltdown thinking that if I appeared to not need her as much anymore, the world would be more likely to take her from me.

And I felt the cancer the day that o2 went out of service for twenty-four hours, which also happened to be the day that mum had her lumpectomy, meaning that I had no contact with anyone or any reassurance that she was OK – thanks, o2.

Now, I just feel incredibly lucky. I feel lucky that I have a mum that's recovered (as much as a person can recover) from a super aggressive form of breast cancer, when it could have so easily gone the other way. I feel lucky that my new flat came with ridiculously dangerous blinds that tripped her over and caused her to check for a bruise on her boob. I feel lucky that it was caught before it had spread all over her body. I feel lucky that Mum got diagnosed in a time and in a country where the doctors are like wizards with magic and potions that can do the impossible. And as I always have, I feel lucky that my mum is my mum.

Love Lauren (Melanie's daughter)

Well, that was an emotional read for me again! This is a poem I wrote…

> 4th June 2019 –
> ONE YEAR ON…*by me.*
> *A year ago today, I was a mother, a daughter, a wife*
> *Then the bombshell dropped and changed my life*
> *Why me? How could this be?*
> *Sorry Mrs Green but you have the 'Big C'*
>
> *There have been many times in life when I've felt a 'right tit'*
> *Now my bloody life revolved completely and utterly around 'it'*
> *Prodded, injected, poisoned, burned, poked some more*
> *OMG I'm going to become a cancer bore*
>
> *Looking like Uncle Fester became my norm*
> *Every day feeling like I'm in the middle of a shit storm*
> *Fatigue, sore joints, the weirdest of side effects*
> *Surgery, mammograms, and on-going checks*
>
> *Ignorance was bliss but seriously, who knew?*
> *I'm just amazed that I got through*
> *Getting back to 'normal' takes some doing*
> *But living to the max is what I'm pursuing*
>
> *And one year on I'm cancer free*
> *Love and laughter have totally helped me*
> *So, thank you so much to those I hold dear*
> *Let's raise a glass and say good-bye, and good riddance, to this year*

16. Love and Forgiveness

This is a bit of a digression from *the* story but it's part of *my* story, so I hope you don't mind this slight diversion. Bear with me, we'll get back to all of the crappy stuff soon.

7th March 2016 –

The 'kids' may both be 'proper' grown-ups now, twenty-five and twenty-three (yikes, surely, I'm not that old) [now 30 and 28!], but I would give my life for them – just as I would have from the second they were born. Any of you who are parents 'should' know that feeling, that overwhelming rush of love when you first set eyes on your baby. And then you have another – how on earth can I love another child in the way I love this one, my heart isn't big enough – oh so wrong! The love doesn't divide, it multiplies, and it is unconditional with absolutely no boundaries.

Of course, there are times when being a parent is hard (haha massive understatement of the century), times when you sit and cry with frustration, times when you cannot wait for your precious little darling to go to bed, go to school, just go! But those feelings are only fleeting, even throughout the 'terrible twos' and the 'terrible teenagers'!

The majority of the time children, no matter what age, bring unbridled joy, fun, and absolute love to those involved in their lives, be it their parents, grandparents, aunts, uncles, and other family and friends. For those of us who are blessed to be parents, and I wish with all my heart that could happen for all those who want it, we should treasure these special gifts with all of our hearts and souls. Now I am sure most of you would think this goes without saying, of course you do this without having to try, parenthood is such a magical and special bond. But unbelievably this is not always the case, not every parent puts the wishes and needs of their children before their own wants, selfishly living life like they don't even exist in some cases. It amazes me that anyone would not want to be fully involved in what their children are up to, to join in the successes, the failures, the fun, and even the sorrow. It truly saddens me that this is the case, but I also can't help but feel a bit sorry for the 'absent' parent – he misses out on so much... so much love, so much joy, so much future, and somehow this alters a lot of the memories for the most precious, amazing, wonderful (I could list 100 adjectives here) people that I know and have the absolute privilege of being able to love with everything I have.

Please, please, please treasure the ones you love, make sure they know how you feel, and know that spending time is the most important present you can give those you cherish.

But just because someone is part of your family, doesn't mean they are good for you –

7th March 2016 –

Should you always forgive even if it doesn't feel right? Now I'm not a religious person (although I do think there is 'something' after we leave here) so I don't feel a pressure to forgive everything or everyone. On the other hand, I also can't be bothered to hold grudges and find it easier to just forget and move on – but does that mean I really forgive, or I'm just too lazy/scared to challenge the hurt? I'm not sure to be honest. Does being able to forgive make us better human beings? Can we really control our emotions and feelings to that extent? Can we make ourselves forgive or do we just think we can and really the things we 'forgive' are the things we are not really bothered about in the first place? Is every act worthy of forgiveness, or are there occasions when Mother Teresa would have to think twice?

I watch in wonder when I see a mother or father, on the TV, saying they forgive the person that murdered their child and I question if they can possibly really mean that? How could they? Do they believe in God and believe that he will have retribution if it is required? I'm quite jealous of people who have faith, who believe everything is God's/Allah's/Jehovah's (for example) will and they have the belief that He has a plan for everyone. It must be nice to take comfort knowing that someone, supposedly, always has your back even though you can't see, touch, or hear Him.

I am definitely a more understanding person as I get older. I like to think I can look at things reasonably, assessing the facts, viewing things from different angles and perspectives. Even during jury service, which involved a child abuse case, I could look objectively at the evidence (wow that was an experience – it was really like a television drama with the prosecuting barrister being the main star). Big G jokes that I'd be rubbish in the police force as I think everyone is innocent…I think that's more about me not wanting to believe that anyone could possibly be *that* evil, *that* calculating, *that* vile. But I know I still couldn't forgive someone taking the life of a loved one – surely despite His plan, everyone has free will to act, and choose their own path, be that good or bad?

7th March 2016 –

And who benefits from 'forgiveness'? That may seem an odd question but bear with me! If forgiving someone makes you feel like you have betrayed yourself and your feelings, should you do it anyway to make the other person feel better? Or does forgiveness make you feel better, even if you are not sure if you really mean it?

So many questions – and I am not sure I am anywhere near closer to having the answer!

So here is my quandary…something happened many years ago to someone I love very much – I won't go into details as it is not my story to tell – but it led to an exchange of texts and emails between myself and another person (who I was very close to at the time) with some vile and, I would go as far as to say, 'unforgivable' things being said about me and about the person at the centre of the issue. Sorry to sound vague but I just needed to give you a little snippet of what happened!

This was four years ago [10 years now] and I have not spoken to this person since then, which in truth hurts because they meant a great deal to me before this happened. However, I never believed they could be so hurtful and cruel and therefore made the decision that I could not trust that they wouldn't hurt me again and so could not allow them to be part of my life. But here's the thing…What happens if this person dies? How will I feel knowing that it is too late to put things right? It is extremely difficult even writing this – I know nothing will ever 'put this right' so what is the point of forgiving? I don't

> *want, nor could risk, this person being in my life so if I open up a conversation, and potentially 'forgive', what will that achieve? Can you lay down conditions with forgiveness such as I forgive you but still never contact me again – but then is that really forgiveness?*

When I got my cancer diagnosis, I contacted this person as I felt they should know. Conditions *were* laid down though…I'm telling you this is happening to me but this does not mean I want to see you…but this person thought they were more important than me, my feelings, and so insisted that they were going to be involved and come and see me. It's like they wanted to come and be 'chief carer', sweep in and make everything better, which of course they couldn't. It was a bit like when someone dies and the whole town takes to Facebook and everyone seems to compete with who knew/loved the deceased the most…who really is the 'chief mourner'! With a few threats of what would happen if this person ignored my requests to stay away, they finally agreed not to come. But I guess that answers my question – no, no you can't lay down conditions, as they don't bloody work!

> 7th March 2016 –
>
> *So maybe you can see my dilemma – if nothing is to be gained from forgiving, as there will still not be any kind of relationship, why bother? To make the other person feel better (I know they feel bad about what happened) but that may, in turn, make things worse for me? Should I be unselfish and do it because I am a 'good' person? Or will making peace help me to put the past in the past? Will I gain a sense of relief? Another*

thing that scares me is if I don't forgive and something happens will I be able to live with the potential guilt of not making peace? But if I only forgive because I am more scared of the consequences of not forgiving, surely that is just bullshit?

I often write things down to help me make sense of a situation and give myself some answers. Well, that didn't work! I think, I hope, that the answers will just come to me one day, maybe something will happen that will allow me to see things clearly, one way or the other, and until then I will just have to forgive myself if I do nothing and the inevitable happens.

I have decided to do nothing with my situation and I am at peace with that. I'm not saying this won't ever change but I really cannot see that happening. Sometimes you have to go with your gut, protect your heart (and the hearts of your loved ones), move on, and deal with any consequences if, or when, they occur.

17. Little Heartbreakers

When I talk about myself and my own illnesses, one thing that's got me through is my ability to laugh and have a joke with it. I can make jokes about looking like a Mitchell brother or Aunt Sally and at many times have even laughed through my tears. This section is about Lauren though, and when it comes to my kids hurting, I don't seem to have the same ability to make light of their situations, so you may notice a slight change of tone in this chapter.

8th April 2016 –

When we give birth, we want their lives to be filled with love, success, and of course good health. We want them to have a better life than ours, to be filled with everything they desire.

I can remember my mum telling me she wanted me to 'be more' than she is. I used to think she was silly as she has a great marriage to my dad, they have a lovely house, she was a teacher (which she loved) and they were reasonably comfortable financially. Why on earth would I not be happy with that as my lot? But now I get it, you want your children to have everything, an amazing family, a beautiful house, a good career, and health and happiness always.

But what if this doesn't happen? How are you meant to feel? Guilty that you didn't do a good enough job? Angry that you couldn't make it happen? Sad that your child does not have a 'perfect' life (but then again what is perfect?)? Frustrated that, no matter how much you wish you could help and take their pain away, there is nothing you can do?

I think all of the above, with many other emotions added to the mix. Watching your child suffering is the worst feeling ever. Not being able to 'fix' the problem is heart-breaking. And not knowing why this is all happening to your beautiful baby is so difficult to handle.

Looking back, I guess Lauren has always lived with a certain level of anxiety. When she was at junior school, her anxiety led her to have a couple of hypnotherapy sessions which gave her the confidence to deal with things and ask for help. But the panic attacks started around the age of fifteen. This meant she hardly went to school, and when she did manage, she spent most of the time in the medical room and I had numerous phone calls to go and pick her up. Then it was the summer holidays, and she hardly left the house, just spending her time watching TV and eating toast! She did receive some CBT at the time, although this did not seem to help (not sure it was appropriately aimed at a fifteen-year-old – there was no bridge offered between what is aimed for children, aged four, and adults, aged forty!). But then, as quickly as they started, one day the panic attacks stopped!

If only that had been a permanent change!

8th April 2016 –

Life seemed to get back to 'normal' for a while. I'm sure Lauren had stuff going on but I was unaware of anything at the time. But then we jump to a few months before her 18th birthday. Lauren is lying on the beautician's table having her legs waxed and I felt a wave of panic wash over me when I looked at her. Now I knew she'd lost a bit of weight, but as a teenager she was very private about getting undressed around me so I hadn't realised just how much she had lost. Her legs were just bones and skin – not the shapely, womanly figure she had developed. I can remember feeling sick to my stomach and had no idea how to tackle talking to her about it. I can't really remember what was said, but I remember feeling that I had to 'fatten' her up before it got any worse.

It was a battle between wanting to force feed her and also not to make a big deal out of food as I thought this could make the situation worse. Every time I went shopping, I was on a mission to find things that would tempt her to eat just a small amount. I was so scared of losing my baby but had to put on a brave face as I didn't want her to feel any of the fear and anguish I was facing. We plodded along for the next few months, she got thinner and thinner but I think I was too scared to take her to the doctors for fear they would diagnose an eating disorder, thus making it real. So, I continued burying my head a bit, trying to get her to eat, and willing her to get better.

Christmas came and went and Lauren went back to school, or so I thought! After a week of her leaving the house at the normal time, and coming home at the end of the day, she admitted that she had dropped out of 6th form before Christmas! I didn't have a clue how to react – my baby was throwing her life away and I didn't know what to do. But then I took a minute and realised that her health and happiness were far more important than her education, and that she could always go back the following September.

Within the next few days, I had a 'lightbulb' moment – maybe she could go to Canada and stay with my family for a few months. This was a crazy idea as neither of us really knew this family (we were talking about my birth mother and the family she had since married into) but I was getting desperate. Nothing I was doing was helping Lauren get better so I thought maybe a complete change of scenery would be the answer. I knew it was a 'do or die' situation, literally, but what other choice was there.

I jokingly suggested it to Lauren, who immediately sent an email to Lesley in Canada, and within a couple of days her flight was booked, passport ordered, and she was leaving in three weeks. Looking back, it was a very brave move, for both of us, but I have no doubt it saved her. I still feel guilt and shame that I couldn't 'save' her (after all it's my job), but also proud that I had the courage to let her go. But in the end, it doesn't really matter what, or who, helped her through that awful time – just that she got through it.

Sometimes there are no reasons for the shit that happens...but unfortunately sometimes there are as I found out.

I spent the week after she left in tears. I remember doing a supermarket shop and bursting out crying in the middle of an aisle.

For months before she went, my main focus when shopping was buying things to tempt her to eat, suddenly she wasn't there to look after anymore and her recovery was out of my hands. Then I started crying even harder, realising that she was alive and had a chance now and others weren't so lucky. I know this sounds a bit dramatic, but I felt lost and desperate!

I needed to feel close to her, so I decided to clean, tidy and sort her tip of a bedroom out, so it would be perfect for when she got home (which was not for another six months!). Tucked at the back of one of her drawers was a folded piece of paper addressed 'Mum'. So, I sat down to read. A cold feeling of despair took hold of my entire body as I continued to read – Lauren had written about the experience that had happened when she was thirteen and I knew nothing about it (it is her story so I won't share more about what happened). I screamed for Big G to come; he ran up the stairs wondering what on earth was wrong. I just passed him the letter, as I couldn't talk due to shock and tears. As he read, I could see his body slump, wtf, how could this have happened to Lauren, and how could we not have known?

But what could I do about it? Lauren had only been gone a week of a six-month trip. Should I ring her, email, skype? How was I meant to talk to her about this other than face to face? Should I jump on a plane? But how could I? She'd gone to Canada as a last resort so how could I jeopardise her recovery? Having discussed it with Big G, my sister, and my best friend, it was decided that I would keep it to myself until she returned home. I'm still not sure that was the right decision but you can only do what feels right at the time. It's fair to say it was the longest 6 months of my life, for many reasons! Sometimes I wish Lauren had had the confidence to talk to me about what had happened before this, but I'm so pleased that she managed to do so eventually. Since then, I think she has shared everything about what happened with me. I know she worries about me getting upset, but she knows without a doubt that I would always rather know how she is feeling. I don't need her to protect me – I'm the mum, I'm the grown-up – I can deal with everything she needs me to deal with, and will be there by her side (even if I can't help that much or make it all go away).

We don't know for definite that this experience, at thirteen, triggered her mental health issues, but they have certainly had a major effect on her life. If only we could turn the clock back...

I so wish it didn't but unfortunately the 'story' continues...

15th August 2016 –

One of the main, and most recent manifestations of Lauren's anxiety, is agoraphobia. Looking back this has been an issue for many years but last August [2015] it took over her life. She was unable to leave her flat, therefore unable to go to university (she actually only managed to go to one lecture in her entire last year but through her determination she graduated this July), unable to travel home, or even go to the corner shop. Now, many people believe that agoraphobia is a fear of open spaces, a fear of leaving your house...this is incorrect. Agoraphobia is a fear of not being able to escape from a situation and therefore 'sufferers' are unable to use public transport, be on a motorway, travel over a bridge, go to the cinema, visit department stores, go in a lift, even use a cashpoint machine...well you can't just leave half way through a transaction. Due to anxiety, and typically having panic attacks, a person's 'safe zones' decrease and they find themselves confined to their home – and this is when we would normally hear about someone having agoraphobia, hence the misconception.

Alongside misconceptions, there are plenty of misunderstandings as to how to 'get over' agoraphobia. I find it difficult to explain to others how it is for Lauren, which is not surprising as I don't always get it – I'm not sure she even does 100% of the time! Last year, when she was at her worst, I used the following analogy for my sister (a very concerned Auntie who really does just want the best for Lauren) who was struggling to understand why she couldn't motivate herself to go to uni, to come home, to go to the shop, and why setting goals did not make a difference, no matter how much Lauren wanted them to. The pain she feels, the struggle she faces, is like someone with two broken legs being told they have to climb Sacre Coeur (which has a tight spiral staircase with 270 steps). I was trying to get her to see that although we all know that it is the mind that causes anxiety, and panic attacks, the symptoms and pain are as physical as any other illness and therefore she can't just 'think' herself better, in the same way someone with broken legs can't! I think the analogy finally made my sister realise that it is not a case of mind over matter, thinking positively, and just pushing through it, and no matter how much she wants to be 'well', some things are beyond her control.

At times I have wanted to shake Lauren to get her to see what she has going for her. I have definitely shouted at her, got arsey with her. And if dragging her onto a train by her hair would help, then believe me I would be willing to do it. I was telling a friend the other day that if I could do anything to make Lauren better, even if it meant she never spoke to me again, then I would do it in a shot (as I'm sure any parent would). But these are in my moments of desperation... desperate to see her live her life to the full, achieving everything she wants, and having a happy life. But if I'm being totally honest, I guess it is for selfish reasons as well. Lauren and I have such a good relationship and we love spending time together. We can laugh at situations that no one else would find funny, take pleasure in the little things, and are just generally the best of friends. So, I miss her! I still love curling up and watching a film, cooking a meal together, coming up with mad business ideas etc. [definitely still do this]. *But I miss going shopping, having meals out (whilst watching coaches go past with naked people having sex on them...a very random experience whilst out for a meal in Headingley!), and would love to be able to go on holiday with her and Kieron sometime. But most of all I miss seeing her happy.*

Lauren is now doing amazingly well but can still struggle with daily tasks that the rest of us take for granted. She pushes herself to do more all the time, and strives to help anyone with anxiety live an easier life.

15th August 2016 –
Talking about mental health is imperative in order to raise awareness, reduce stigma, and to ensure those living with issues know that they are not alone.

18. Sticks and Stones

We need to remember that language and our choice of words can be far reaching and damaging in all aspects of our lives. Ill-considered comments about someone's appearance, personality, family, health, etc. can have long lasting effects.

20th September 2016 –

Sticks and stones may break my bones, but words will never hurt me! What a load of bollox!

Saying the wrong thing to someone can damage them forever. A flippant, throw away comment that is meant to be taken light-heartedly may impact on an individual either because of how they are feeling that day, or because of something that has happened to them in the past... The problem is that you could say something one day and it would be fine, and another day it could be taken badly or be hurtful. You may also never know the consequences of your words as not everyone will break down, cry, or scream, but instead hold onto it, internalise it, allowing it to affect them deeply. So how do we get it right?

Unfortunately, there is no magic list of phrases, no magic formula. When I was away doing some mental health training a couple of months ago [2016], I kept asking for a list of what not to say but was told that learning to say the right thing would come with experience! Great, so they expected me to experiment with the use of language on individuals living with serious mental health issues – not ideal! The consequences could be devastating. But I also know, from personal experience, that they were right and you just have to try to get it right, and always admit and apologise if you get it wrong.

I think the best advice I can offer about talking to someone who has mental health problems, and anyone else for that matter, is to take their lead. If they use certain words then it is probably OK for you to – but again you can always double check with them.

Just ask…questioning how the person would like you to talk about any issues they may have, the words they would like you to use, will not be offensive – this will just show you care. Also, don't say nothing in fear of getting it wrong. Saying nothing feels like you don't care, and I would much rather have a fumbled attempt of saying the right thing, then be sat across from someone and wondering the whole time, 'do they even care what's going on with me right now because they don't seem like they do?'

> 20th September 2016 –
> Also, let the pace they may want to communicate about anything be set by them, don't push, don't expect answers, and more importantly don't expect miracles – talking is fabulous 'therapy' but it will not heal everything. Just being there to listen will go a long way though, so always take the time to do so.

Talking about mental health issues will not cause suicide, but not talking about them might. Easier said than done I realise as it's scary to start the conversation, but let the person know you are there and willing to listen to whatever they need/want to talk about, whenever they need/want to talk.

> 20th September 2016 –
> There is a saying – 'It's nice to be important but it's more important to be nice' and this is so so true. Letting the people you care about know that you are there, for ALL of the bad days as well as the good, couldn't be more important. Saying the right thing at just the right time can have such a positive impact on the receiver, and therefore, in turn, the giver of the comment.
> Guess the 'moral' of this post is…if you can't say anything nice then don't say anything at all, always think before you speak but also always

speak with good intentions and from your heart, and try not to take offence if you don't get the response you were hoping for! It is better to try to get it right and sometimes fail (which I am sure I do often!), than never to try at all – that just feels like you couldn't care less!

Don't be embarrassed to apologise if you don't get it right. Sometimes we slip up, say the wrong thing, use the wrong term… as long as it isn't done maliciously, then I'm sure you will be forgiven…but if you don't acknowledge that you got it wrong then it may be too late to undo any offence taken. And that being said, maybe we should learn to tell people if they say things that we find offensive or hurtful – I'm clearly saying do as I say, not as I do…I hate confrontation and have had many hurtful, vicious, nasty things said to me, and about me, and I just take them because…oh I don't know, probably nerves, maybe because I don't want any aggravation, and more than likely because I am a massive people pleaser – often to my detriment.

19. Generosity and Friendship

1st October 2016 –
I am always amazed by how generous some people are with their compliments, kind words, and encouragement. To take time out of your busy lives to a) read my blog and b) send me a message, is just overwhelming.

Wow! If I thought they were generous with their words about my first blog, which this is from, imagine how overwhelmed I felt once I started telling my cancer story a couple of years later.

1st October 2016 –
When I started this blog, I felt very embarrassed about sharing it with 'the world' but I have had so many expressions of support that I feel truly blessed. I caught up with a friend in town this morning who said I have a way with words, which is such a compliment. I have never kept a diary, never written stories (well since school – and the only one I remember was a blue/rude one...the English teacher made me read it out in class! I think he was trying to embarrass me – he succeeded! I wish I'd kept it!), and although I have just finished my degree, academic writing is obviously very different. When I write my blog posts, I just let the words pour out of me, trying very hard not to edit as I go, and hopefully this comes across when you read them. Hearing that people are relating to my experiences gives me a huge boost. Knowing that by reading my blog, some of you feel that you are not alone in what you're feeling and going through, is just amazing and inspiring. It makes me believe that opening up my heart and sharing my feelings, thoughts, and insecurities, is completely worth any embarrassment I may feel.

So, this is just a short post to say THANK YOU so much for your interest, your kind words, and your thoughtfulness.

Again, wow! I need to keep reading this old blog post as I am writing this book. So many friends have said I should write a book, that I've got a book in me, that I should share my experiences. But then you look on the internet about getting a book published (there's a proper task for another day) and you read that it's nigh on impossible, and just because people tell you that you can write, that they relate, does NOT mean you can, or should, write a book that anyone will want to read, or publish, or that it will sell. To be honest I try not to think that far ahead whilst doing this…I just let my ideas flow (if I can remember them) and try not to edit my thoughts as I go. If you are reading this then Thank You, if not, then you won't care less!

7th October 2016 –

Friends are the family we choose. There is a saying that people come into your life for a reason, a season, or a lifetime. I believe this is true for all relationships, but especially when talking about friendships.

Reasons could include emotional needs, guidance and support, as well as physical needs. I'm trying to think of friends that have featured in such a role in my life and although I am sure there have been some, I'm struggling to pinpoint one!

I would love to be one of those people who still has the same circle of friends now that I had at school but this is not the case for me. I still 'know' a couple of the girls I was friends with as a teenager but only really on social media. Life moves in different directions I guess and maybe school was a 'season'.

This has changed since my cancer diagnosis. My best friend at school was Allison – the one that was always late! Boyfriends, jobs, life, meant we drifted away from each other. When our children were young, we saw each other for play dates but then we drifted apart again. We were 'friends', happy to know about each other, commenting on each other's photos when Facebook came along, knowing a bit about each other's lives, but not really about each other in detail. But when I messaged to tell her about my diagnosis she jumped in, always knowing what to say, asking questions, making coffees, giving me some normal times. Luckily Allison can talk, non-stop (soz), but that was amazing…when I wasn't feeling great, she talked, I listened – thank you.

> 7th October 2016 –
> *I would like to think I have many friends but if I'm truly being honest (which I promised you I would be) then I would have to admit that most of them should really be classed as acquaintances. Would I feel that I could ring them at 3am to discuss my anxieties? Do I believe they would drop everything to come and make me smile when I'm feeling down? I'm afraid I would have to answer no to these…maybe because I wouldn't feel comfortable asking them but there must be a reason for that!*

Again, since my diagnosis, and now with Covid-19 and isolation thrown in the mix, I think that has changed. I now value all of my friendships and just because I couldn't call at 3am (more my issue than theirs), they definitely make me smile. And just because we don't see each other regularly (a lot of that is down to me because I am actually a rubbish friend and am dreadful at keeping in touch – luckily those that want me in their lives know that and 'excuse' me for it), I do know that they are there for me, as I am for them.

> 7th October 2016 –
> *BUT I do believe I have one such friend who I will have for a lifetime, whether she likes it or not!! Having someone who is prepared to share your joy, your sadness, in fact all of your emotions, is a gift and one that I personally cherish with everything I have –* Thank you Kerstey…for being you, for being there for me and mine.

20. Miscarriage and Grief

This is another chapter of my story that doesn't have much to laugh about in it. Life isn't all fun (slight understatement) but I think it's important to share it 'all' – I promised I would!

24th October 2016 –

Miscarriage is the loss of a future, the loss of dreams, the loss of the ability to share your love in the most natural, fulfilling of relationships.

Losing a child is incomprehensible and no one should ever have to bury their child. Although miscarriage means you don't physically get to hold your child, from the second you are pregnant you can imagine your arms around them, loving them, protecting them.

The word 'miscarriage' in itself conjures up the idea of failure. Applying the prefix 'mis' conveys doing something wrongly/badly (misapply/mismanage/miscarriage of justice). So, does this increase the idea that you are a failure? One in four pregnancies end in miscarriage or stillbirth. We need to open up and talk about this subject so people do not feel alone in their grief and know that they are not at fault.

Let me tell you my story...

Eight years ago [14 now – wow we'd have a teenager] *I was sick in a bush whilst out walking the dog sparking crazy thoughts that maybe I was pregnant! I already had two children who were aged fourteen and sixteen at this point from my first marriage. I was now with Big G and we had decided not to have another family as he also had a daughter from a previous relationship. To say the thought of being pregnant was a shock is an understatement! But I was. In that moment, it was very scary, and we talked a lot about whether we should continue with the pregnancy. In truth, initially Big G thought of it as a problem but I couldn't help that I had already fallen in love with my baby.*

> *We went to the hospital for a dating scan to enable us to make a considered decision. It was there, sitting in the waiting room, that the realisation hit Big G. This wasn't a 'problem', this was a baby – our baby. I could visibly see the love enter his heart. But then our world came crashing down. Our baby had died, there was no heartbeat and so the medical procedure was booked in for a few days later to take my baby away.*

Lying in hospital after being given some pre-op drugs, I remember thinking they had made a mistake and that my baby MUST be alive. I couldn't be going through this, it wasn't fair. At this point it felt like I was the only person in the world going through this pain, feeling this grief, but obviously I wasn't – too many women/men/families experience this, too many times. I wanted them to redo the scan, but was too afraid to ask and in reality, I knew there was no mistake.

> 24th October 2016 –
> *The doctors were lovely and reassured us that we could try again for another baby – but I didn't want another baby...I wanted THAT baby, MY baby. I don't think I've ever cried so much, howled even. I felt physical pain in my heart with the yearning for my child. I was 'only' ten weeks pregnant but the grief I felt was just so intense. Having thought about it since, I think the grief must be about losing the future with the child that you already feel a real, and everlasting, love for. From the minute you realise you are pregnant, consciously or unconsciously, you begin to plan and dream about this baby, this child, this adult.*
> *The support and love I felt from family and friends were amazing, although I had to tell them first that I had been pregnant and in the same breath that I wasn't any more. I'm not sure the 'modern' idea of keeping pregnancy a secret until after the twelve-week scan is a good thing. If anything happens, you (or I did) need people to understand the*

> *pain and despair you feel. And if they didn't know about the pregnancy in the first place, then they are not invested in the process and may brush it off with such sayings as 'something must have been wrong', 'it wasn't meant to be', 'nature's way of dealing with problems', and other dismissive statements. I call bullshit!*
>
> *Again, being totally honest, this is how I was before it happened to me. I used to sympathise with people who had miscarried but I didn't really 'get it' and understand the overwhelming grief someone can feel. Now I do. I'm not sure why I had to go through this pain but I have to believe that it was another experience that gives me the ability to understand and truly empathise with others going through the same thing, having walked in those devastating shoes.*

Just on a selfish note, how many devastating shoes can one person walk in! Enough already – I don't need to experience everything shit in life to make me understand/empathise/be a good person, or a good listener!!

But as with cancer, everyone's 'story' of miscarriage/pregnancy loss is different. No one's story is worse, no one's story is easier, just different. Just because I have been through it didn't really help me comfort Lauren when she went through a molar pregnancy. I still didn't know what to say, or know how to help. But she knew I was hurting for her, and for myself to be honest as I fell in love with the baby the minute she told me she was pregnant, and hopefully she knew I would have done anything to take the pain away.

> 24th October 2016 –
> *I know I'm one of the lucky ones as I already had two beautiful children, and for that I feel blessed, as many people are unable to have children.*

94

21. I Just Want to Look Like Someone...Anyone

18th May 2016 –
Several of my life experiences led me to choosing psychology as a degree, one of which being that my daughter, Lauren, lives with mental health problems. But I think one of the main reasons was the idea of nature versus nurture as I was adopted as a child and was fascinated about the concept of whether your genes or your environment have the most influence on your personality.

It is always difficult to answer the questions about family medical history. I had some details in my adoption papers but they obviously only covered details up until they were filled out – and didn't cover any new illnesses my birth family may have developed in the following years. More unanswered questions!

18th May 2016 –
A little bit of history...My birth parents were fifteen and sixteen when I was born and in 1970 girls were 'forced' to give their babies up for adoption, which is basically what happened in my case. So, when I was ten weeks old, I went to live with my Mum, Dad, and sister Bryony (who is also adopted but never had the same need to know her history – everyone is different and there is no right or wrong way to feel about this stuff). And what a happy childhood I had. I can't remember being told I was adopted; I just seem to have always known. I was free to look at my adoption papers whenever I wanted and being curious about where I came from, I did this fairly often.

Apart from when I was very young, I have always been very open about the fact that I am adopted. Some people are ashamed; some people are embarrassed; some people just don't even think about it. With all personal journeys, much like how I feel about dealing with cancer, there is really no right or wrong way as to how to feel, act or cope with the situation. Granted, it was easier for me having had a happy upbringing with very open and supportive parents. Now don't get me wrong, I haven't been walking around openly introducing myself like, 'Hi I'm Melanie and I'm adopted' but if the subject comes up then I am always happy to talk about it. My children always knew but one occasion when we talked about it in depth was when Connor, my nephew, was born by caesarean.

'Did we come out of your tummy?', they asked.

'No, you came out of Mummy's special hole!!'

'Did you come out of Nanna's tummy or her special hole?'; this was the start of Lauren and Kieron's real understanding of what the word 'adoption' means. There have been many times with the children in our family when we've realised that knowing the term 'adoption' and knowing what adoption actually means are two very different things. This conversation was when that changed for us and resulted in the comment, 'So, you've got two mummies then Mummy?';

'mmm I guess so'.

Years later, Connor discovered that Bryony was adopted (I think he would have been about 6 or 7) – he was very upset that Nanna wasn't his 'real' Nanna and Kieron wasn't his 'real' cousin – clearly not bothered about Lauren also not being his real cousin!!! Haha. To be fair, Kieron was, and still is to some extent, his hero!!

18th May 2016 –
I had dreams that my birth mother was a fairy tale princess with a long flowing dress and one of those tall pointy hats with streamers flowing down her back (I have just Googled it and the headdress is called a hennin. Always learning!). I still held that image into adulthood. If I'm honest I didn't really think about my birth father growing up, not sure if that is because I'm a girl or if that is the norm for most adopted children. When I was eighteen Mum said she would do anything she could to help me look for my birth family if I wanted but I was not at all ready then.

More than wanting my birth mother to be a princess though, I really just craved a person in my life that actually looked like me. Everywhere I went, I could see family resemblances between brothers and sisters and parents and children, and that's not something that I ever had. I wanted it so much that I think this is in part what made me want to have children so early. I'd always wanted to be a mother, but I also really wanted to have some biological family in my life, and not because 'blood is thicker than water' (because let me tell you, it isn't!) but because I wanted at least one person in this world to look like me. Then someone could say 'wow, hasn't she got your eyes' and actually mean it. And so that's what I did, I had Lauren.

18th May 2016 –
I was twenty-one when I had Lauren, and twenty-three with Kieron. Two perfect babies who looked just like their dad (annoyingly!).

Lauren came along with bright blue eyes and tight curly ringlets much like her dad. In fact, there was no resemblance to me at all! And then came Kieron, who looked so much like his dad that he used to assume photos of his dad were actually photos of him! I remember a friend jokingly asking why I had Graham (ex-husband – yes, I clearly only marry Grahams!) sitting in a trolley in the supermarket because Kieron was the absolute double of him! There is a theory that babies look like their dads when they are first born so the dads know the baby is theirs and therefore are more likely to bond quicker. In theory the mother's identity is indisputable; however mine looked so like their dad that I did begin to wonder if I was involved at all!

18th May 2016 –
How can this be – I still didn't look like anyone! Now this may sound strange but for an adopted person I think this is quite a natural feeling. There is no 'oh don't you look like your sister', or if there is then you just look at each other with a wry smile knowing they have just said it once they found out you are related – this happened to us a few times. And for some reason, looking like someone is important!

So as the years went on, they still didn't look like me (Lauren does now though). My curiosity continued to grow to the point where I spoke to my sister about looking for my birth mother on a drunken night out in October 1999. I still hadn't plucked up the courage to talk to Mum and Dad about it, which was silly, as I knew they would be behind me 100%.

Although I knew this, and we had talked about it since my 18th, I still didn't want them to think they weren't enough – they were more than enough, the best parents ever. The other thing that stopped me was not wanting to disrupt my birth mother's life. I mean obviously I was scared of being rejected and having the door slammed in my face, but I was more scared of rocking the boat that was her life. I couldn't know if she had told people or if I was a secret. I absolutely, and unconditionally, had no malice towards her. I knew that she had written to the adoption society when I was about a year old to see if I was ok…my dad replied with the loveliest letter as you can see below…so I knew she hadn't abandoned me, she had no choice, and it was totally the best thing for me to be adopted.

'My wife and I have heard through the Children's Society that you have been unhappy and worried about little Rachel [my name that my birth mother gave me].

My dear if you could see her at the moment sitting on my wife's knee with her sister, listening to their bedtime story, you would understand at once that she is happy and secure as a toddler can be. And we both love her as much as a baby can possibly be loved. Do try to put your mind at rest. Rachel will never lack for anything that we can possibly provide and that certainly includes all the love and security in the world. She is a very sweet little girl and we are profoundly grateful to you.

God bless you and send you peace' – How amazing were my parents?!

18th May 2016 –
But then the weirdest thing happened – on the 20th January 2000, I received a letter from the society through which I was adopted, saying they had information about someone who may be a relative of mine!!

First of all, I thought it was a scam of some sort. They would tell me we were related and then need money or something. But all day it kept gnawing away at me…what if it was legit? So, I dug out my papers and that's when I realised it was from the same organisation that arranged the adoption – the Church of England Adoption Society.

> 18th May 2016 –
> *Once I rang them and he* [the intermediary at the adoption society] *had established that I knew I was adopted (that could have been a major revelation!) he told me that my birth mother wanted to get in touch with me! OMG! Only three months after I had decided to look for her – spooky!*

I'm not sure how hard it would have been for me to look for Lesley, my birth mother, as she had moved to Canada and married. She had to do the search through an agency (the only legal way) and it only took them 1.5 office hours to find me, so it obviously wasn't that tricky even after almost 30 years had passed. I guess I'd only moved to the next county and only married once (by then!) so I wasn't that much of a mystery! For some people the search is not that easy, and some never find the person they are desperately searching for.

> 18th May 2016 –
> *Apparently, she had been waiting since I was eighteen for me to come looking and because I hadn't, she got fed up of waiting! (Oops – I think she's forgiven me for my tardiness!) The intermediary told me that she lived in Canada, had a seventeen-year-old son – I had a brother – and I still to this day have no idea what else he said as I think I went into shock. I rushed round to Mum and Dad's and just handed her the letter...*
> *'Oh that sounds interesting', she said*
> *'Mum, it's her, she wants contact', was my reply!*

Christos, my brother, didn't know about me until Lesley had instigated the search, a few months before I was 'found'. Her husband, Thom, and some of his family knew but that was it. I totally understand her reasoning for not telling Christos – she didn't want to give him the 'green light' to do whatever he wanted through his teenage years...'Well, you had a baby at fifteen' may have been thrown back in her face! Luckily, he was happy at the thought of having a big sister and embraced the situation.

18th May 2016 –

Now let me say this – my Mum and Dad, and my sister, are the most amazing people on this planet. Where many people would feel threatened and jealous about this new development, they all embraced the idea and couldn't wait to thank my birth mother for having me and allowing them to raise me. If that isn't one of the most unselfish reactions, I have no idea what is.

Emails and phone calls, trips to Manchester where Lesley was from, and I was born, to meet the rest of the family, and eventually in the April [2000] she came over from Canada to meet me...my life was in a total spin for months, years even. But I still didn't look like anyone...

The first time I met most of the family in Manchester (I'd already met my grandmother, Lesley's mum Shirley, a week or so before) I felt like a monkey in the zoo. I was sitting in Shirley's house and every time an uncle (four of them!), aunts or cousins arrived they just seemed to stare at me! But at the same time, I was staring at them, trying to find a resemblance, trying to see that I now looked like someone, but nope. They all looked alike but still not like me. Due to my social anxiety, the only way I knew how to deal with this gathering was to get drunk, very drunk. I tried to keep up with my 'new' Auntie Julie – big mistake! As I tell my stories I'm always a little embarrassed at how many involve too much alcohol!

Comparing photos of Lesley at the time I was born (she was 15) and Lauren at the same age, there is definitely a similarity that I can see now, but I still find it difficult to see one between myself and them. When Christos saw pictures of Kieron as a young child, he thought they were old photos of him too, so there are more family similarities. I've always found it strange how genes work and that you can really look like multiple people at the same time; in that Kieron can look so like his dad but can also really look like my side of the family, to the extent that photos can be mistaken for the same person on both sides!

18th May 2016 –
    Fast-forward to 2003, and you will never believe this but, my birth father came a looking! I won't go into too much detail but just to say that one of his daughters looked like me – finally. And as for the nature versus nurture debate, well I was so like him in personality it was uncanny. I firmly believe that I get my morals, manners, and to some degree outlook on life from my wonderful Mum and Dad, but there is no denying that genes play a major part in the formation of your personality – it was once said that I was my birth father in a dress!

My extended family proves that blood/genes aren't everything. In the past I wanted to do a family tree but was always put off not knowing which family to focus on. In recent years Lauren got someone to do hers, therefore mine, through the bloodline, so my birth family. She decided to do this after we commissioned someone to look into Mum's family tree and even though nobody in those findings were blood relatives, we still found it fascinating because this was still our family, our family's family, and where my Mum came from. Now having a biological family tree too, this has been fabulous to look at and I now know so many more pieces of my puzzle than I ever thought possible.

Families are very complicated though and parts of my biological family are estranged, so again proving that blood is not thicker than water (well it is, but you know what I mean). In terms of my adoptive family, the family tree is very far flung. One of my aunties, Dad's sister, Auntie Meg, fostered a lot of children, and those that were around my age were brought up as cousins, which they still are. Bryony and I weren't the odd ones out in our family – not many of our generation are actually blood related, or even from the same heritage, making our whole family unit a wonderful mix that 'chose' to come together and stay together. Another of Dad's sisters, Auntie Jenny, has a big family party each year and it's sad to think we will probably lose touch in many ways when she no longer does these. They say you can't choose your family, although we were chosen for ours, but I would still choose mine anyway! One of the reasons Lauren wanted to do the family tree was to see if she had a bit of something different in her genes, be from somewhere/anywhere other than England…shame it revealed her whole family (mine and her dad's) are only from Manchester, with a bit of Norfolk and Suffolk thrown in – which is weird as that is where we ended up!!

The reality of meeting up with your birth family does not always lead to happily ever after – like it seems to in films and on the TV. There are often deep-rooted feelings and emotions involved – lots of guilt, anger, bitterness about missing out/ abandonment, expectations not met, etc. but I am very happy to know where I come from, fit the missing bits of the jigsaw, and look like someone. If this resonates with you, and you want to go looking for your family, just do it with caution and realistic ideas about the results. My family is, and always has been, the family that I grew up with and I always was, and continue to be, eternally grateful for that.

22. Relationships

Relationships change and transform naturally over time. Life-changing events can destroy or have a positive effect on a couple and I was very fortunate that our relationship grew stronger after my diagnosis – Big G was my absolute rock.

> 26th June 2016 –
>> *How do you keep the spark alive?*
>> *I am still amazed (and shocked if I'm honest) that, after thirteen years (19 years now!), I still want to spend time with Big G, don't want to murder him when he's eating a biscuit (well not much), and that I love him more every day. This has never happened to me before, with my longest relationship being eleven years, which were six too many!*

This 11-year relationship was with Lauren and Kieron's dad. We were together for three years when we got married and Lauren was six months old, and Kieron came a year after. The breakdown was not really anyone's fault – I think we just grew up and grew apart. It was my decision to finally call it a day. The children were nearly seven and nine and it was then or never, as I was considering the effects on the children once they were at high school and in their teenage years etc. It was certainly not an easy choice as I took my vows very seriously and planned to be married forever. I know some people thought I was being selfish and not thinking about what was best for my children. But I, 100%, know that it was the right thing…for us all. A few months after we separated a customer's mum came into the hair salon I was working in. She was telling me that she'd been married for almost 60 years…

how amazing, that's just what I'd planned when I married – er no…she'd been miserable for most of those years. But life in the 1950s, when she had young children, was very different and it wasn't possible to leave. Wow, if I hadn't been separated already, I'd have left that day! Life is too short to be unhappy – or too long depending on how you look at it!

26th June 2016 –
Obviously, compatibility is massively important but I have to say opposites really do attract as me and Big G couldn't be more different – I am 'highly strung' (for want of a better term – I'm sure he would call it something different!) and if Big G was any more laid-back he really would be horizontal!

This has changed a bit over the years…he gets more agitated the older he gets – he may still end up under the patio yet!

26th June 2016 –
But I also think you really have to work at a relationship and although it is wonderful to be comfortable with your partner, you have to make sure 'comfortable' is not another word for 'bored'!! So, I have compiled a few ideas to keep the spark alive and have fun in your relationship…
During the course of a relationship one person, at any one time, will make more effort than the other. This is natural and doesn't have to be the same person all of the time, it can swap around depending on what is happening. If you feel like you are the one that is always making the effort, remember this and try not to get frustrated and angry. Sit down with your other half and tell them how you feel and work out ways to alter this. I can remember one couple I knew and it was always the wife that made the effort, arranged nights out, sorted the kids etc. She used to get very upset that he never arranged a babysitter or made

any sort of effort to treat her, and in the end, she stopped trying as well. He wasn't a bad person; it just didn't come naturally to him and he was quite happy to chill at home. As I was a friend to them both I did try to give him a nudge in the right direction with a few ideas. The main suggestion being to set an alarm on his phone, say once a month, reminding him to do 'something', be it arrange a night out, cook a meal, or even just tell her that he cared! Not sure he could be even bothered to do that but it really is worth a go, and very easy to do, if you find yourself being 'lazy' and slipping into not making an effort! It may seem a bit calculated but better to set a reminder and have a happy partner in my book!

Date nights are such fun so why wouldn't you!? Spending the day sending flirty texts in the build-up to the evening, planning what to wear, even pretending you are on your first date and playing games where you ask questions about each other – you may be fabulously surprised by the answers. These nights can involve going out, staying in with a take-away, or cooking a romantic meal together...light the candles, put on your heels (guys too if you want!), put your slap on, and treat each other to some quality time, perfect.

Re-reading this just made me think of a night out in Edinburgh. You often see scenes in films where couples pretend not to know each other in a bar and chat each other up; anyone in the bar would think they were strangers. I think we had even discussed this earlier in the day. Big G was showering in the hotel and I got it in my head that this would be a fun thing to do – I had clearly already been on the wine! So, I quickly got dressed and went down to the bar, ordered myself a large glass of wine and sat at the bar trying to look sexy!! Eventually, he came downstairs and straight away said something like 'oh there you are. I wondered where on earth you had gone'…not quite the chat up line I had been hoping for!

26th June 2016 –

Write a love letter...or even just a note, and leave it on his/her pillow, in a lunchbox, write it on the toilet paper! Such a tiny act will make their heart melt – trust me!

I am obviously still waiting! Big G is the kindest man, worships the ground I walk on, supports me with everything I do, but romantic, in the traditional sense, erm nope!

26th June 2016 –

Be spontaneous! Not always easy with everyone having busy lives but it will be well received and totally appreciated...However, I am still waiting to find a new dress laid out on the bed with a note telling me to be ready in an hour as he is whisking me off for a romantic evening!! Not sure I should hold my breath for that one as I have hinted so many times, and when I say hinted, I mean told him so many times that I would love for that to happen! Haha.

…still waiting!!

26th June 2016 –

Kiss...a lot...and for no other reason than you want to!

Time is one of the most important things (although clearly diamonds and presents are also greatly appreciated so, please feel free to spoil me if you are reading this Big G!). Make time for each other, even if it is catching up over a cuppa at the end of the day for a five-minute chat. And don't use having young children as an excuse. Believe me when I say they will grow-up so quickly, and even before they leave home, they will not need you in the same way, and then what?

And last but by no means least...say 'I love you' often, spontaneously, when it is least expected, but never out of habit!

Relationships need work but if you put the effort in, the rewards are immeasurable.

23. Is Validation and Approval from Others Really Necessary?

2nd July 2016 –

Is anybody reading this? Does it matter? Do I care? These were questions I discussed with Lauren while we were out for dinner and a few drinks last night.

Does it matter? Not really, although I'm not sure I like the idea of being a sad, lonely, middle aged (do I really have to admit this) lady who is full of her own self-importance and naivety, or pretentious enough to think anyone would bother to read my thoughts, rants, moans, and dreams! But then if no one is reading this then at least I've found somewhere to express these ponderings – and on a positive note no one will see that I have just admitted being middle aged!!

Do I care? No should be the answer, but if I'm truthful then yes... yes, I do care. Why? Is it because I believe I have something worthwhile to say? Maybe! Or is it because I have so many insecurities that I need some sort of validation for most things I do? This is the more likely reason! The majority of people I meet believe I am the most confident person, but this is all a front. I spent far too many years 'sitting in the corner' but as I grew up and had my children, I came to realise that this would never get me anywhere and so I learned to 'be confident' on the outside whilst sometimes crying on the inside. If people really get to know me then they can see the anxiety I live with on a daily basis, and although it doesn't usually stop me doing anything it is a real and exhausting sensation.

About two months after starting a new job, one of my colleagues said to me, 'You are actually really nice. When you first started work it seemed like you thought you owned the place and I didn't really like you. But now I know that isn't the real you and you were overcompensating.' Summed me up right there!

Anxiety has often stopped me going to social events, especially on my own, even if it's just drinks round a close friend's house. I always get a nervous headache/stomach ache before going out, even if it's just for a meal with Big G – it infuriates me but hey, I just have to try and ignore it, paint a smile on my face, pull up my big girls pants (maybe pop a couple of paracetamol), and crack on.

24. Do You Tell Your Hairdresser Everything? Having an Outlet to Vent

Having someone, anyone, to talk to about the bad, the good, the ugly that is happening in our lives is so important. I am very lucky to have an amazing family and wonderful friends, who I can share my deepest fears with, along with my happiest and proudest moments. But not everyone is so fortunate or wants to talk to their nearest and dearest about certain topics – so sometimes you have to find this outlet elsewhere.

> 6th August 2016 –
>
> *How have you been since I last saw you? A phrase that often seems to open the floodgates as any hairdresser will tell you! The styling chair appears to be as powerful as a therapist's couch.*
>
> *I was a hairdresser until earlier this year [2016] and I have lost count of the number of times I was asked for advice and listened to clients reveal their most personal thoughts, which often included a fair amount of tears.*

Sometimes these customers followed my advice – OMG please don't do that; I have no idea what I'm talking about!!

> 6th August 2016 –
>
> *It is accepted that we 'tell our hairdressers everything' but have you ever considered why? Well, I have...and even did my dissertation for my psychology degree on aspects of this, really quite odd,*

relationship and the sharing of secrets, thoughts, feelings, and advice seeking.

One idea is the intimate element of the relationship between hairdresser and client. Touching is a necessity when washing hair, cutting, and colouring etc. The washing process usually involves a head massage (and before my old clients shout at me, I know I was fairly rubbish and lazy about this), not to mention the client's face being in close proximity to my armpits and boobs whilst leaning over them – not such a pleasant experience, I'm sure! And throughout all of the practical tasks, personal space is continuously 'invaded'! This could be quite intimidating if it were not for the friendly and easy-going nature of the hairdresser. Relationships are built over time and this then provides a safe place to discuss personal issues.

A person's appearance is extremely important as to how we present ourselves to the world. Therefore, having trust in your hairdresser is essential. So, does this trust transfer to what you talk about? If you trust them to make you look 'fabulous darling', would it follow that you would trust them with your secrets? It is a unique relationship that is only really comparable with maybe beauty therapists – you see them every six weeks or so, can spend hours sitting in the chair, and because of the chatty, sometimes annoyingly so, personalities of hairdressers, you WILL talk to them whether you like it or not!! There is nothing worse than a client who wants to sit in silence, but I did have to accept it sometimes and tried not to bully them into opening up (too often)! Friendships evolve, but as the hairdresser you are not usually involved in clients' personal lives and this may be another reason why...who are you going tell? You don't socialise with their family or friends (although I often did – lots of weddings which was so lovely), and they trust you, so seems a natural progression to reveal all!

I also think there may be an aspect of self-reflection in the exchanges. Whilst you are sitting in the hairdresser's chair you are constantly looking in the mirror with the hairdresser behind you, so are you just sounding off and actually talking through your issues

> *with yourself? Sometimes when we ask for advice, we already know what we want the answer to be, deep down. We just want someone to confirm that our decision or feeling is right! It is like tossing a coin... it doesn't help you choose which way to go, because if it lands on the 'tails' when you wanted 'heads' you start playing best out of three!*

So actually, maybe it does help – if the coin doesn't give you the 'right' answer first time, maybe you have your answer – and had it all along! I think we should listen to our instincts more. We doubt ourselves so much – not sure if it's more about worrying what other people will think about our decisions more than us worrying we are going to 'choose' wrongly – I know I am very guilty of that. Have the confidence to 'do you'...you are your biggest cheerleader, your loudest advocate, but unfortunately you are also your ultimate critic...stop that cycle of self-doubt now!

> 6th August 2016 –
> *Being someone's confidant and having people open up their souls to you is a real privilege, one that I was always in awe of, and I know things about my clients that nobody else knows, even their closest family members, and I will take what they have told me to the grave.*

In fairness this was a two-way thing...my clients knew everything about me and mine. Many times, Big G would be in the kitchen (next door to my salon), listening to me reveal all sorts – why on earth would she be telling them that?! He got used to it in the end, didn't really have a choice! I'm a heart on sleeve and open book kind of a person! Which is just as well or this would be a very short, boring book!

25. Waiting Is So Frustrating

> 1st November 2016 –
> *Whether you are waiting for a bus, a flipping boiler man who promised you he would be here yesterday (yes, I am cold and haven't had hot water for almost 3 weeks but luckily, he has turned up this morning or I'm not sure I would be able to control my anger!), or waiting to hear back about a job application, you keep checking your phone or the doorbell to make sure it works!*

I'm not sure waiting has ever been more painful than waiting for a cancer diagnosis (or any life-altering illness) for yourself, or your loved one. The days seem endless, the nights more so. When you are waiting you think it's the worst thing in the world – knowing would be better than this, at least then I can deal with whatever the outcome is – mmm, until you don't have to wait any longer... then that's the worst thing in the world!

> 1st November 2016 –
> *As you can probably tell I am having a frustrating week!*
> *Four years ago, I embarked on an academic journey that I am still amazed by. A few years previously I toyed with the idea of going to university and applied to do psychology but my application was declined as I had been away from education for so long. I left school at sixteen, and when I say left, I mean I practically ran out of the door, down the road, and never looked back. I hated school and just wanted to be out earning money. I did a few office jobs before having my children, then a few part-time jobs until I decided to retrain as a hairdresser when Kieron went to school – I was twenty-eight! But*

years of cutting and colouring hair made me miserable. I absolutely loved the social aspect of the job, hearing people's life stories, their troubles and their worries, that part was a massive privilege and so the idea started to form that maybe I could retrain as a counsellor and so university beckoned again.

After spending a year completing an Access to Higher Education course, I obtained a place at the University of East Anglia to do a BSc in Psychology. Who would have thought – little old me doing a degree? I was forty-three at this point, clearly never too old! Three years of travelling five hours each contact day, up to four days a week, and still doing hairdressing in the evenings and days off, I GRADUATED! What a hard journey, many tears of frustration and self-doubt, but so many laughs with Katy, Katie and Ollie – many times wanting to throw myself 'under' a bridge! And yes, I know that wouldn't hurt too much but that's as brave as I get.

So back to my new career path...I changed my mind regarding counselling and decided I wanted to help people who lived with mental health problems in a more practical way. To my amazement I got one of ninety-six places, on a graduate programme in which 2337 people applied, to train as a mental health social worker – I know!!!

Six weeks of intensive, residential training, with only going home for one weekend, took its toll, but I was determined this was the career for me. But four weeks into placement I had to make the heart-breaking decision that I wasn't strong enough to do this. I am not sure if such self-awareness is a good thing or not – if I wasn't so aware maybe I could have carried on but I know it would have ruined me in the end. I am not one to sleep well at the best of times, but the reality of this job was too much for me. The potential consequences of me not doing my job properly (which is a real possibility with the caseloads and lack of funding) could be devastating and I witnessed this within these first weeks. Therefore, four years, six weeks away from home, and four weeks commuting three hours a day and observing the most amazing people working against the odds, I had to admit to myself, my family, my friends (although I haven't told many people yet, until now, due to embarrassment) that I could not do this.

> *To say I'm disappointed, ashamed even, is an understatement. I know it was a brave, and probably, wise decision – the few people who know so far have said all this to me – but now I'm lost. I have been so busy for the last four years...and now nothing! I now need to find a new direction but really want to do something with the knowledge I have gained and still want to help people. I am a firm believer in everything happening for a reason and so I can only hope that the reason becomes clear sooner rather than later and my dream job is just around the corner.*
>
> *I am now waiting to hear if I have secured an interview for a pastoral role within a high school, which I think I could be good at, hopefully! Therefore, I will mainly be refreshing my emails and checking my phone for missed calls all day...whilst I sit in the cold with three workmen fitting a new boiler! If both are successful, I will be celebrating this evening with a hot shower...it's the simple things!!*

I didn't get this job – their loss! I did get a better one though, in a college, working with young adults with learning difficulties. Maybe not directly related to my degree but it certainly helped when I became a team leader and had 17 staff to manage – practical psychology!

As you go through life your goals and aspirations change, well mine have – more than once! So now I'm 'retired', or am I a professional writer? Haha! After the last few years, and with the ongoing health issues we've decided to de-stress our lives and concentrate on having fun – travelling and spending time with our family and friends.

26. Dreams Really Can Come True

Focusing on what is important, and following your dreams, becomes even more pertinent after you receive a life-threatening diagnosis. But don't wait until then – work towards making your dreams a reality every day. No matter how big or small they may be, your dreams are meaningful to you so keep on keeping on.

2nd July 2016 –

When I say Fred Flintstone what comes to mind? A cave man hopefully or this 'riddle' doesn't work! And I have my very own 'Fred' in the form of Big G! No, he doesn't wear an animal print shirt, nor does he say 'Yabba Dabba Doo' (very often!), but he is a carnivore and you regularly see him chomping on a big lump of meat, and more importantly he lives in a cave!!!! Well part time, and I guess, this in turn, makes me his 'Wilma'. A cave you ask... (well you probably didn't but I will explain anyway!) ... yes, a cave, in Spain, built under the ground, a bit like a Teletubby house.

For many years we, like many others, have fantasised about owning a house abroad and have viewed many over the years. A friend, Cathryn, calls us bogus house hunters and says there are probably posters with our mugshots on, warning estate agents that we will waste their time, haha! But nothing felt right, it wasn't the right time, they were too expensive, too much of a risk...always an excuse. So why now? Well, a lot of the reason is the actual cave – location, price, and more importantly it felt like home. But it was also 'well, why not now?' Life is short, and definitely for living – I know so many people who have died far too young and it makes you reconsider your life choices. Why keep waiting...waiting for retirement, waiting for the 'right time'. When is that? How do you know?

It will always feel risky when you do something outside your comfort zone, and I can assure you buying a cave in Spain feels risky (not because we worry about the actual purchase but there is always the worry that we may not use it enough or may regret it) but risks can be fun, as well as terrifying! I used to do a lovely lady's hair and she and her husband were renovating a cave house, which was the first time I had ever heard of them. I loved seeing the pictures as it progressed, and the plan was to retire in five years' time. Well only about a year after starting it, they thought 'bugger it' and retired early to go and live their dream. We lost touch unfortunately, this was in the days before Facebook, and recently I found out that she had died about two years after going to Spain. This really affected me...what if they had waited five years as originally planned? She would never have got the chance to experience the life she dreamt of – scary thought. I am so pleased they went early and I really hope she had a brilliant time. So just do it...take a risk, make your dreams come true.

Earlier this year I read 'Driving Over Lemons' by Chris Stewart, the original drummer with Genesis, in which he and his wife bought, and renovated, an old finca in Andalucía. This made me even more determined to make our dreams come true – if they could do it why couldn't we? The problem is that it has also makes me want to renovate something (the cave doesn't need a lot doing to it) so the question is... what next? An almond farm maybe...

It has also made me want to write a book, 'Flaming Tomatoes', one day maybe...one dream at a time! [Maybe one book at a time, eh?!! Next year, who knows!!]

We have just arrived back from 'Cueva Contento' (happy cave) [2016] and it was such fun having new furniture delivered, sitting in front of the log burner, designing terraces on which we will be able to admire the fantastic view whilst sipping a vino tinto, and making our cave into a home...here's to many years of happy cave dwelling...Yabba dabba doo!

Unfortunately, circumstances have kept us away from our piece of paradise but we will get back there soon…it is just waiting for us to spend more time there. The last few years have definitely proved my point – why wait? And what on earth are you waiting for? You need to grab any bit of happiness you can get. That may be a cave in the sun, a boat, a tent, holidays, new sofa, or a new plant for your garden… everyone's happiness is different, and everyone's happiness is valuable and worthwhile. Help your family and friends achieve this happiness if you can – the joy they get from it will 'repay' you tenfold.

27. Christmas is the Best Time of Year

As I've mentioned before, I could be classed as a 'little' bit of control freak when it comes to Christmas. These are a few of our 'must dos', or at least they were before cancer made me reevaluate what is actually important!

> 1st December 2016 –
>
> I have always been, and hopefully always will be, a massive fan of Christmas. I even love the stress of running around last minute making sure everything is ready – however my family may not 'love' the 'stressy' me!
>
> We have quite a few family traditions (although when I say family it is mostly Lauren and myself as the 'boys' don't really get in the spirit!), which start early December and end on Boxing Day and I thought I would share a few with you.
>
> The first weekend in December is tree putting up time. Lauren and I like to put it up early as I am a bit of a 'bah humbug' and want the tree down as soon as there are no presents under it! So usually the day after Boxing Day (and it has been known on Boxing Day itself) the tree comes down and we get the house back to normal, ready to see the New Year in. So the first weekend in December we play Christmas songs and make the house look like Santa's grotto and this sometimes involves a trip to the local woods to find a 'twig' that we also decorate for the dining room!

When I say find a twig…it is a full scale, covert operation. We only ever take one from the ground, so one that has already fallen off a tree and dead. But sometimes they are too big…so we go armed with a couple of saws, (as Big G is not the keenest of DIYers these saws have seen better days and would have trouble cutting through butter, never mind a branch!), and spend time finding just the right twig with lots of extra little branches for decorations to hang from. The saws are always hidden under our jackets as we feel that we may be judged as axe/saw murderers! Then comes the struggle to get it into the car, hoping that no one sees us (unlikely when it's a very popular area for dog walkers) as there is still the feeling that we are doing something wrong. Then it's home to spray it, and usually most of ourselves depending on the wind direction, a hectic scramble to find something to put it in, and finally the fun bit – lights and decorations. Once we even made a last-minute cardboard star when we couldn't find one in the ten minutes before the shops shut. We're not very good at waiting until the next day to finish it off, it has to be done right there and then.

1st December 2016 –

We also have a Christmas baking day when we make apple and sausage rolls (yum), mince pies and anything else that takes our fancy! This year I even made one of the desserts for Christmas day as it can be frozen – very organised!

Miracle on 34th Street – a **must** in the lead up to Christmas! And this year we are seeing it live at a local theatre! Soooo excited!

A new tradition I want to start when I 'eventually' (haha, no pressure there then) have grandchildren is to make Christmas Eve boxes including things like new pj's, a Christmas film, and other goodies. I've already 'informed' Lauren that this is something I want to do for them, and I will inform Kieron's other half when the time comes! Not a pushy 'Nonnon' at all!

I am Nonnie, not Nonnon, and have kept to my word and started this tradition – I love doing it.

1st December 2016 –
On the day...
For breakfast we always have bagels with bacon and Philadelphia.
I am not sure how that tradition started but if we have them at any
other time of year it always feels like Christmas!

Nowadays we like to mix it up a bit – Eggs Royale or even pancakes and fruit. Who says traditions can't be tweaked?

1st December 2016 –
When the children were little, I was a bit of a 'sergeant major' and insisted on the whole day being 'fun' – nothing worse than 'organised fun', which clearly never turns out to be much fun! So, the routine was opening stockings in bed with me watching – only one present at a time so I didn't miss anything – mad, I'd bloody wrapped the things! Then shower/bath and get ready for the day. This used to involve getting 'dressed up' but now it usually involves putting a clean pair of pj's on! Then it was breakfast before being allowed a present from under the tree. I tried very hard to space these out, to prolong the 'fun', only having one present each an hour, and each person opening in turn so I could watch their faces – it's no wonder Kieron has a bit of a phobia about opening presents in front of anyone! I really am more relaxed now, honest, and have come to realise that our Christmases may not be the 'funnest' or the most 'perfect', but we all have our own 'perfect' and ours involves chilling, eating and drinking far too much, and most importantly spending time together. And if things don't go to plan, so what! 'Memory days' my sister calls them – the ones that go wrong are the ones you always remember and still laugh about years later.

I have become so much more chilled in recent years. Christmas 2018 was only a few weeks after my lumpectomy and reconstruction, so I had to let Christmas happen around me a bit. Lauren put all the decorations up while I watched from the sofa. I still managed to prepare the veg on Christmas Eve, just had to be sat down to do it, and the day was very relaxed. We played Uno, Frustration, and Monopoly; and having my kids and Big G there, with me still being alive, was the best thing I could have wished for.

1st December 2016 –
Because I still want the presents to last a bit longer (I absolutely love giving gifts – in all honesty I'm not worried about receiving any, although it is lovely!), I also buy table presents, which I 'sneak' onto the table so the family are surprised to get another present! After doing it for years I don't think it is much of a surprise but I still like to believe it is!

Charlie has his own tradition of ripping up all of the wrapping paper, even taking the presents out of our hands because he gets too excited waiting. He really is such a good boy though, as the presents are all under the tree already and he doesn't touch them until we start unwrapping.

Our gorgeous Charlie, our Labradoodle, died in 2020 so Christmas isn't quite the same anymore without him there to rip up the paper.

1st December 2016 –
We have two Christmas days – the 'real' one at home and then another at Mum and Dad's which is usually on Boxing Day but happens whenever we can all get together. This started when the kids were little as it was a bit overwhelming to get so many presents in one hit, so we exchange presents with my sister and family, along with Mum and Dad on this very special day. I am very grateful for being able to spend this time of year with my family, many people are not able to do that for numerous reasons. Christmas is a wonderful time of year but remember to treasure your loved ones throughout the year as we never know what is around the corner, and we should not take tomorrow for granted.

Never a truer word written!! Little did I know when I wrote this that 'tomorrow' was very doubtful at times!

28. Big G, The Big C and The Alien

Seven weeks of tests, seven weeks of waiting, seven weeks of despair, seven weeks of tears, seven weeks of hope – life can be a massive ball of shite sometimes.

And then came the diagnosis in October 2020 – Big G had High Grade Large B Cell Lymphoma – totally devastated.

Seven days of thinking the worst, seven days of not being able to look to the future, seven days of fear.

Then we see the consultant (the only time I was allowed to go with him due to Covid-19) and we find out it is aggressive but curable so that's what we tried to focus on. Lots of leaflets, books, emergency number cards, details of treatment, appointments for a bone marrow biopsy and PET scan to see if the cancer was anywhere other than the lymph nodes in his neck…information overload.

And so, the merry-go-round started again, at high speed! Chemotherapy started two weeks later. This time it was very different – I couldn't go with him and support him as he had done every time with me. This was difficult for me, more than him, he's a brave soldier and luckily not a freak about needles like me. Although since chemo he's a bit more wary of them as his veins aren't as good as they were. It is not easy to obtain blood or insert a cannula anymore, so he is definitely apprehensive and sweats, a lot, if they need more than one attempt!

Another big difference was the shielding. During chemo, and for months after, your immune system is shot to bits, so Covid was very dangerous for him. That meant we had to go into hiding for the foreseeable, only going out for medical reasons (it felt quite exciting when we could leave the house) and the odd ninja walk

– it was a very long winter. We are very lucky that we still quite like each other. Lockdown was very tough for many people and couples, but when you literally can't go out you have to set your mindset to comprehend that – difficult but we are still married so we got through it!

Big G was reasonably lucky with his side effects – not as many weird 'surprises' as I had, thank goodness. He got very tired, still does at times, so he would have a nanna-nap every afternoon (thinking about it, maybe that's what saved us being cooped up with just each other for company!) and his sleeping patterns were all over the place. He had neuropathy in his fingers which was very painful sometimes and still is. He lost some of his hair but only the brown bits…the grey hair was super resistant and kept on coming, very annoying, and his bowel movements needed a bit of help!! TMI!

So, there we were plodding along quite nicely and a day or two before his fourth chemo session he had a call from his consultant. His initial PET scan had shown the cancer was in his stomach and spine, so now he had to have six sessions instead of the four we hoped for. Now here's the thing that annoys me most about Big G (OK, OK, there are many things, but at this time this was the worst!), he doesn't ask any questions (I know I have said I don't but I'd have at least asked what that meant). He was now thinking that it was not just in his lymph nodes, but in his actual stomach and spine; however on googling it I found out that you have lymph nodes throughout your body. My thought was, as they weren't changing the treatment and were just extending it (they had warned us this would happen if the scan showed any spread), it was still 'just' Lymphoma. We still don't actually know the answers because, guess what, he still hasn't asked! If we could have gone to a face-to-face appointment, instead of them all being over the phone, I could have asked the questions but hey, that's how it was.

The consultant was still positive about the prognosis though as the lumps on his neck were responding well to the treatment.

Six sessions of chemo, then seven weeks wait for another PET scan to see if the chemo had wiped out the cancer, a further two weeks before the results – which were to be given over the phone. Two and a half hours after his appointment time they finally rang (busy clinic and we'd both rather they were looking after the people actually starting/going through their treatment – but by God, it was a long wait). As I'm sure you can imagine by now, Big G wouldn't put the phone on loud-speaker so I just had to watch and wait for an answer. His first response was to burst into tears, then apologise for getting emotional about the news…. '…er WHAT NEWS? Shit news? The worst news? WHAT THE HELL IS HAPPENING?' It felt like a good two minutes before he finally gave me the thumbs up, but in reality was probably only thirty seconds – long enough when you are waiting to find out if your husband is going to live or die!

Lots of tears then…Big G didn't stop pretty much all evening; after a few tears I couldn't stop smiling all evening. Phone calls and texts to let everyone know the best news ever, phew.

And so I ask the same question again…did I really have to walk in the shoes of cancer to be able to support, understand and empathise with Big G. He did a pretty good job of doing those things for me without experiencing it first-hand! But now I also knew it from the other side – what he had been through: the fear, the helplessness, the wanting to take the disease away from your loved one.

So, what now? Life…travelling…holding my family close. 2020 and 2021 have been the shittest years yet…losing Dad, Big G's dad, April (Lauren's baby), cancer, 'Bob' the brain tumour to name but a few…surely it can only get better!!

I guess I should say a bit more about Bob the brain tumour/Alan the alien (name is a work in progress – suggestions on a postcard

125

please)! In 2019, not long after I'd finished radiotherapy I was diagnosed with Vertigo. Whenever I lay down the room would spin and I felt like I was going to fall over – weird experience as I was already lying down! I was given medication (prochlorperazine) and it stopped after a couple of weeks.

In October 2020 it happened again, but this time it was different in that it was happening when I was sitting and standing, and I had to literally get on the floor because I was scared of passing out (I've only ever really fainted once – at a Simply Red concert at Wembley. We'd rushed up after work, I hadn't eaten, and two songs into the support act I slid down my ex-husband and landed on the floor. We tried to go outside for some fresh air but the door men insisted I went into the medical bay behind the stage. There they tried to get me to drink tea with lots of sugar, yuck, and eventually allowed me to go back to watch the show…but only by sitting in the disabled bay at the back of the standing area. OK, at least I got to sit down and the area was raised so I could still see the stage. I felt really poorly but we couldn't leave as we had left my friend Tina, near the stage, with one of our friends from Felixstowe, who she'd never met! But at least I wasn't going to miss the concert…well until everyone that was in wheelchairs got up to dance…scammers!!).

Back to the vertigo…more medication from the GP; however it didn't seem to improve. And then one afternoon the left side of my face went numb…er, what on earth was happening? I promptly rang the doctors. I was feeling a bit silly, thinking whatever was happening was due to stress as this was at the time we were waiting for Big G's diagnosis, so after telling the doctor my symptoms I told her I was sure I was being a paranoid freak as I was worried I might be having a transient ischaemic attack (TIA). Once you've had something like cancer, you know it is possible for shite things to happen, and it's very difficult to not panic a little. By then the numbness had worn off and I felt OK, apart from the dizziness but she referred me to the stroke clinic at Ipswich Hospital. Within a day or two I had a video consultation, which involved me walking up and down, holding my arms in the air, and answering lots of questions. Nope, not a TIA but due to my history he thought it was sensible if I had an MRI scan just to be on the safe side. This is another 'bonus' of having had a cancer diagnosis – the doctors are always keen to refer you in case the cancer has returned.

One of the ongoing side effects of chemo is the damage to your veins. My body has never been that keen to show my veins when needed – I think my fear of needles makes them disappear the minute they see one coming – but chemo has made this even worse. This made the MRI scan (brain scan) such fun and it took five attempts (ouch), and two nurses, to locate a vein to inject the contrast dye in. This was not ideal as I was part way in the tunnel, couldn't move, couldn't really hear, was crying my eyes out and couldn't even wipe the tears away due to the cage over my face! Based on the fact that it's been over three years since I finished chemo, I'm not sure this situation will get any better – a lovely, ongoing reminder of the joys of cancer!

Lots of tears and trauma – and more to come…

A week or so later the consultant from the stroke clinic rang me. Interestingly (his words, not mine – really not interesting at all, bloody horrifying more like), they had found a benign infratentorial brain tumour (an Epidermoid cyst), also referred to as 'Left Epidermoid filling the left Cerebellopontine angle – with a mass effect (pushes) on the midbrain' which they think possibly caused the numbness and imbalance I experienced. It is surrounding the Trigeminal nerve (CNV) which is responsible for relaying pain, touch, and temperature sensations from the face to the brain and, therefore, could also be the cause of my twitching left eye, swimming eyes, and headaches. The stroke clinic referred me to Addenbrooke's hospital.

I then had to tell the family! As Big G was already having chemo at this point, we were shielding, so I stood on Kieron's doorstep to tell him. I then called round to Lauren's and we went for a socially distanced walk around her estate.

'I've spoken to Addenbrooke's today', I started.
'About your heart?' (more about that in a minute!)
'Er, no, thought I'd try a different department this time'.

My kids are the best and handled the news like absolute troupers, and then apparently, exchanged very inappropriate jokey texts that evening! Always the way we deal with things! I actually feel satisfied that every time I had a bad headache, and tried to get sympathy by saying I might have a brain tumour, I actually did…so I should have had the sympathy I deserved…still don't get it though!

The tumour measures 3.2×1.5 cm, which doesn't sound that big but I'm fairly sure we don't have large open spaces in the middle of our bloody brains, and especially not in *my* highly intelligent brain! And having seen a picture of the scan recently, it looks bloody massive and terrifies the bejesus out of me! These tumours are pretty rare, only accounting for 1–2% of intracranial tumours – I like to be different! They develop when cells that should have become skin, hair, and nails (epithelial cells) become trapped during the neural tube closure as the brain develops.

The specialists at the Neurotology and Skullbase Clinic at Addenbrooke's Hospital believe this tumour has been growing since three-four weeks gestation and the hope is that it is very slow growing. I was scanned again in June this year (2021), luckily without dye this time so it was not as traumatic. Although after being in the tunnel, with the face mask on for about twenty minutes, the operator brought me halfway out and said he just wanted to double check about the dye (I think he must have been surprised with what he saw). He then left the room for what must have been ten minutes and my crazy mind had him forgetting about me and eating his lunch somewhere! There was no change to the size of the tumour. So now I will have yearly MRI scans and if there continues to be no change, this may go to two or three yearly scans. Surgery will not be considered (thank goodness) unless it grows or starts causing me more problems.

It is a very strange feeling knowing I have this in my head. It can't explode (bit dramatic!) but I could get infections in it and obviously if it grows, and it starts pressing more on certain nerves, it could cause further complications – but for now, I try to put it to the back of my mind (or the bloody middle to be more precise) and just try to get as much sympathy from my family as possible – zero chance of that happening!

Lauren suggested the name Alan the Alien because apparently when you go into a room and can't remember what you went in for, you actually see an alien and they clear your mind so you don't remember seeing them! My memory is so bad so we joked that maybe that's what actually happens. But then we realised that I really do have an alien in my head – a 'foreign body' that shouldn't be there!

And just because cancer and brain tumours aren't enough…

There is a close family member who has dilated cardiomyopathy (a disease of the heart wall) which can be caused by a mutation of genes. These mutations can be inherited and I was therefore referred to the Clinical Genetics and Cardiology departments at Addenbrooke's Hospital [approx. 2016]. My consultant, in the genetic clinic, is not convinced that the particular genes identified are solely to blame. They do not want to test my genes in case they show a negative result/no mutation and send me on my merry way, and then I still develop the condition. Although the testing of my genes is in constant review, as the science is ever evolving, we may get to the stage that they are happy to do the test to look for mutations.

A lot of people don't know they have the condition until it is quite far-gone and causing a lot of problems, so finding out early will be a great bonus. Therefore, they check me every year with a 24-hour monitor and an echocardiogram (ultrasound scan), with an MRI scan every three years – how lucky am I to be looked after so well? I do get some palpitations (ectopic/extra beats), which have also been picked up on the monitors so I now take beta blockers (bisoprolol) to limit them. Another big thanks, NHS. But if that could be it for the illnesses, I'd be very grateful!

29.   Did She Really Just Say That?

> 12th April 2019 –
>
> So many friends have asked me what is the right, or wrong, thing to say to someone with cancer. I don't think there is necessarily a right thing – although I try to live by the theory that it is better to admit that I have no idea what to say rather than say something that might hurt someone. That being said, I still think something/anything should be said rather than nothing at all!

It's funny reading this again. When Big G was diagnosed with lymphoma you would think I would know what to say having been through cancer myself. Nope, still no idea – but I followed my own advice, 'I really don't know what to say!'

> 12th April 2019 –
>
> But there are many wrong things that you can say! However, I am very aware that a lot of these comments come from embarrassment, fear of getting it wrong, wanting to offer comfort, but unfortunately some definitely come from ignorance!
>
> Here are just a few of the things said to me:
>
> 'I can empathise with you as my mum had breast cancer'. At this point I'm thinking arh that's nice, and I'm sorry to hear that, but then 'oh but she is terminal now as she has a secondary brain tumour' – er not really what I wanted to hear a day or two after my diagnosis.
>
> Several people have told me the story, 'My mum/my best friend/my aunt survived after having breast cancer three times' – again, not really what you want to hear when starting treatment for the first time!
>
> 'Will you survive?' Erm, not sure how you answer this one so my response was simply 'I bloody hope so'. This is a weird one because

> *I think most of us would like to ask this question when we hear of someone with a cancer diagnosis but social etiquette means we don't – but it still totally took me aback!*
>
> *Another strange one is 'Your positive attitude got you through this'. Now I really do appreciate these sentiments, and I absolutely know they come from a good place. However, I feel it somehow diminishes the 'struggle' people who haven't survived have gone through. I'm sure they all started out with positive attitudes but it didn't help them. I feel 'lucky' to be alive and doing well – but then I feel chuffing 'unlucky' to have had to go through this in the first place.*

I know I've mentioned this before, so I'm sorry if I'm repeating myself, but a lot of the 'language' used in relation to cancer... warrior/war/battle/fight... win/lose/brave...are metaphors that some people find motivating. That is fabulous for them but they make me feel uncomfortable; they are just not for me. I wasn't brave; I didn't have a choice but to do as I was told. I wasn't a warrior; I didn't have a choice but to do as I was told. I didn't fight cancer; I didn't have a choice but to do as I was told. It's only the cancer that determines who lives or dies, who 'wins' or 'loses', no matter how hard you 'fight', no matter how 'brave' you are.

> 12th April 2019 –
>
> *And these were said to other cancer patients who I have had contact with:*
>
> *'It is much worse for your husband watching you go through the treatment' – now I know it is very difficult for loved ones to watch someone go through it, but I'm still fairly sure it is worse, much, much worse, for the person actually having the poison pumped in, the surgery, the intense burning of radiotherapy, and all the other little gems that cancer brings!*

Now seeing it from the other side, I agree, it was incredibly difficult watching Big G go through his treatment. But I still stand by my statement – it was much worse for him in those moments, than it was for me!

12th April 2019 –

A lady returning to work after treatment –

'Have you been on a sabbatical?'

'No, I have had cancer.'

'Goodness, you don't look like you have had cancer' (Umm, not sure what I should look like). Then...

'I know just how you feel I had to have a long-time off work but it wasn't cancer' Well I don't really suppose you know how I feel then!

A lady who went to a cancer support group who'd had bladder cancer was telling another lady, who was recovering from breast reconstruction, that breast cancer was best because you can have your reconstruction and then forget it!

On hair loss: 'Your hair was very thin anyway!' – I couldn't quite believe this one! That's ok then. I mean why would you be upset about losing it then...never mind that it means you have bloody cancer.

This next one may not be an inappropriate comment but I loved hearing it, and it properly made me laugh – 'I call what's left of my breast 'Robin', because I love robins and I'm delighted to still have my red breast!' [It was red from radiotherapy].

This is just a very small snapshot but it may just make us think a little before we jump in and say something potentially hurtful. I can laugh at, or brush off, most comments, but a few have left me speechless. However, I can say terribly inappropriate things but having a sense of humour (most of the time) has got me through this, so that is my excuse! It's not just me though; family and friends have been known to shock a few people with 'near the knuckle' comments!

Big G with the news of my diagnosis, in front of the consultant and breast nurse – 'I will remarry, you know' – his way of saying don't you dare die as I have always said that I will haunt him if he finds someone else!

> *'Cancer take me now!', at a party with the most depressing music on – lots of people there I didn't know, oops, well this is me!*
>
> *When shopping with a friend, 'Oh no, I couldn't possibly pack the shopping as I have cancer!' – not sure the lady on the till knew what to say!*

Big G and I continue to make inappropriate comments – who has had the 'worst' cancer experience and who has the most serious ongoing health issues…. But I think I can play top trump now with the brain tumour (and I do use that too – 'Oh, I can't possibly, I have a brain tumour…!').

> 12th April 2019 –
>
> *We tend to make light of things and I'm sure the stuff that we say to each other could really offend someone else. So, this post can only ever be from my perspective – I find things funny that others may struggle with. On this point, I have noticed on Facebook that many people get annoyed/offended when someone shaves their head to raise money for cancer research, saying things like how can this help, how can they relate etc. I'm sure none of those people think they can understand how a cancer patient feels when losing their hair, and how the feelings are tied into this hideous disease, but I still think it's a pretty brave thing to do… shame none of my friends wanted to come out in sympathy and shave their heads!! Well apart from Charlie, our Labradoodle, who went a bit bald on his back at the same time as I lost my hair (this was unfortunately due to testicular cancer which was luckily sorted with a quick op)! And in all honesty, I think anything that raises money, and awareness, should be praised. A friend's daughter, Hope, is shaving her hair off after she completes her GCSE's this summer – hats (or hair) off to her.*

She raised £2500 for Teenage Cancer Trust, and also donated her hair to the Little Princess Trust, and I had the pleasure of doing the shave – it wasn't emotional at all!

30. The Menopause or is it?

The menopause (mine was medically induced with the Zoladex injections, a preventative measure to help stop the cancer coming back) has brought me lots of little joys that I was not expecting. This little gem that all women have to endure, although some breeze through it (lucky cows), is quite rightly being discussed more and more on the TV – because the misunderstandings and misgivings about it are massive, and it can be life changing and devastating for some women!

I thought I should google menopausal symptoms and there are so many. But OMG, so many of mine could be attributed to other conditions (cancer, heart, brain tumour) that now I really don't know what to put everything down to! Not that it matters but it makes me realise I haven't got much chance of avoiding a lot of the joys, and apparently cancer can increase the severity and duration of the menopause – thanks again cancer!

So here are a few of my symptoms –

Hot flushes…about twenty a day! I think the sweaty neck, under my chin, that accompanies them is the worst! I've been lucky that I've only had one or two night sweats but it's still covers on, covers off, feet in, feet out, all flipping night.

I am oh so forgetful and struggle to focus – but is that the menopause/chemo brain/brain tumour/age…who knows? I have to write things down the second I think of them, or they're gone! And as for remembering places we've visited…literally no recollection of some things/places at all. Big G jokes that he's going to tell me one day that we've already been to Hawaii (my dream destination ever since I was young – well surely Magnum will greet me off the plane with a lei and whisk me off in his Ferrari...not that I'd be able to get out of it now!) because I can't remember where we've been so this will save him lots of money – cruel!

Poor sleeping/insomnia – to be fair I've always struggled with this. My mind does not shut off, if anything it gets more active as soon as my head hits the pillow. I get very cross with Big G when he goes to sleep instantly...well surely that's what you are meant to do when you go to bed, he says! But now I have the added joint pain and sore boob, so getting comfy is an issue. I'm getting to the point that I'm going to look for a travel mattress topper anytime I'm not in my super soft bed!

Weight gain/difficult to lose weight – now is this down to the menopause or the amount of shite I put in my mouth?

Low libido – who can be bothered with all that messy business and not helped by the dry fanwah...bit ouchy (soz for the TMI, again!).

Extreme fatigue and tiredness – definitely better than straight after chemo but still hits occasionally so is it now due to the menopause? Or is it due to the other condition I have...lazyitus?

Itchy skin – OMG this actually started to drive me mad. My back was constantly itchy and the lack of movement in my shoulders after surgery, that lasted a couple of years, did not help the struggle. Definitely invested in a back scratcher!

Chin hairs! As I'm so dark haired I've always had a tash, but I'm not loving the chin hairs! When I was about 14, I remember I shaved my tash off before going on a school trip to Holland. Someone noticed it growing back and I had the pee properly ripped out of me. So, when I got home, I had electrolysis on it, but it was too painful for me. I then bleached it for a while, but a blonde tash isn't much better! I now wax the bugger...as well as the chin. But that's as far as the waxing goes...again way too painful for me.

I remember Kerstey saying she could wax my bikini line without it hurting – what a big fat lie – I made up swear words that day!

Hay fever and allergies – who knew this was a thing? Not me! Apparently when our immune system comes under stress, it releases histamines, which cause allergic reactions. So, because of the intimate connection between hormones and our immune system, it's not unusual to notice some changes to our allergy profile during the menopause. Last year I popped antihistamines daily due to hay fever and thought it was odd that at 51 I'd suddenly start suffering from it but there you go…I'm a bit sensitive anyway as I'm allergic to horses, cats and some dogs so may be more susceptible to this symptom!

Mood swings – now I don't think I'm too bad with these although Big G may say different! I never really suffered from PMS so maybe there is a connection? I know some friends, not mentioning names, who want to stab their husbands at times!

Joint issues/pain, headaches, breast soreness, hair thinning, incontinence, heart palpitations, and osteoporosis in my back (more than likely accelerated because of the Letrozole I take for cancer prevention) are all other symptoms I have but again, these may be attributed to the menopause or the other 'conditions' I have!

Every woman's story is different and support is out there if you need it. Even though some of my symptoms drive me mad, I don't think they impact massively on my life, or maybe I've just learned to accept them. HRT can be an amazing help for some women. This is not something I can have due to my cancer being hormone fed but I would certainly look into it otherwise as I can't really see the point in suffering with something if you can ease the shiteness, even if just a little.

31. My Dad (1934–2021)

You always think your parents are invincible, that they will always be there to love you, support you. My parents have always been that to Bryony and me. We have given them many worries over the years, from Bryony being a nightmare teenager (I could fill a whole book with her exploits!), to her having Connor at twenty-six weeks' gestation and we nearly lost them both, both of us divorced, money worries, health issues, general family stuff…but even if they didn't approve of our choices, our decisions (and they did tell us!!) they were always there for us, and our children.

Growing up we had a lovely childhood. Nothing extraordinary, no massive adventures (well apart from having a boat, Vinca, on the River Deben which I absolutely loved – Bry not so much unless it was stationary! Oh, and having a house cow called Sally when we lived in Bressingham!) but it was safe and secure. Simple memories of Dad making dove noises with his hands (I spent hours trying to copy and never managed it), tricking us into believing he pulled string through our necks, hours of Cat's Cradle (he knew so many sequences and never got bored). Dad developed epilepsy when I was about 8, so things changed from then. He was ill a lot, more than he was well, so he had to retire from teaching early. Mum had to step up to be Mum and 'Dad' – work full time, keep house, do the fun stuff, and the not so fun stuff with us, whilst also caring for Dad – I took it for granted when I was little, and probably for years, but how amazing was/is she, and I love her zillions. Luckily Dad's health stabilised a bit by the time the grandchildren came along and he got to create some wonderful memories with them.

Easter 2021 – he went into hospital on Good Friday; we were told he was very ill on the Saturday, improving on Easter Monday morning but then he died that evening. We were all in shock. He was nearly 87, didn't have the best of health, but he wasn't dying… but he did. I still don't think it has sunk in yet. We had a very quiet funeral (because of Covid, but it would have been exactly as he wanted), scattered his ashes on the river next to our old boat, and now we have our memories and stories. We did have a bit of a laugh during the scattering of ashes…the wind blew and the ashes went all over Mum's trousers! So, Dad still managed to come to the pub with us for his last meal! We now have a memorial bench to visit that looks over the mouth of his beloved River Deben.

Dad was so intelligent and well read (he even read the Indian Times online) and could remember the most random facts. He was involved with Google trials and ran an Apple bulletin board, having self-taught himself all about computers and programming, before most people had PCs. My Dad was the most gentle man I've ever met.

Love you forever Dad xx

32. Have a Lifesaving Fondle

23rd October 2018 –

As I'm sure you are all aware, October is Breast Cancer Awareness Month. I think it is brilliant, but come November I'm fairly sure the prompts to check our breasts will soon get forgotten – not even sure I bothered in previous Octobers to be honest.

So, I just wanted to stress the importance of getting to know your boobs, and yes that means you too men – they are not just there to admire...although admiring and getting to know your partner's lady bumps can only be a good thing as I know someone whose husband found her lump. All boobs are different, unique, and it's about getting to know your own. Both of yours could be a different shape, size, and density, each nipple can be a different colour, shape and size – so what you are looking out for is CHANGE...because it might just save your life...and that's the power of love – oops sorry, felt a song coming on!

You do not need to get obsessed about checking, once a month is perfect. For pre-menopausal women, it is best to check a few days after your period. Your monthly cycle can affect the feel of your breasts and some can become very lumpy around the time of periods. This is quite normal, which is why it is suggested to check them post period. For post-menopausal women, and for men, put a date in your diary, set a reminder in your phone (and don't ignore it), for example the first of the month, and make that your regular check day. It is still vitally important to do this even if you have mammograms as some breast cancers, like mine, can be very aggressive and unless timed perfectly, your next mammogram may be too late to pick up symptoms in time for early diagnosis.

There is a lot of information on the internet about how to check your boobs so check them out if you aren't sure. However, these do not say about checking lying down as well, which is just as important as I pointed out in a previous post about finding my lump. I couldn't feel it standing up, even though it was quite large. However, I may have noticed changes if I knew my boobs, as underneath there was large indentation so if I had looked at my breasts in the mirror, with arms above my head, and checked from every angle, then I would probably have seen a CHANGE!

Here are a few stats: [correct at time of writing the blog post]

1 in 8 women will develop breast cancer in their lifetime and 80% of these will be over 50 years of age. Scarily one person is diagnosed in the UK every 10 minutes, which equates to about 5,000 each month, approximately 60,000 a year! This compares to 370 new cases of breast cancer in men per year, showing how rare it is...but you still need to check yourself!

Early detection and diagnosis are vital as 90% of women survive at least five years when diagnosed at the earliest stage of cancer, compared to around 15% surviving for the same amount of time when diagnosed with the most advanced stages of the disease. With this in mind, when you notice ANY CHANGE, something that is not normal for you, please, please, please, book an appointment with your GP immediately. I know how scary this is, but remember that nine out of ten breast lumps are benign – not cancer!

I'm just hoping that this post will encourage you to firstly get to know your boobs, and check them monthly – if this can make a difference to just one person then you will make my day, month, year.

There are many resources online, and in the media, with information on checking and being breast aware. CoppaFeel! is one such charity and, as I mentioned them before in this book, here is the website address for their online resources:

https://self-checkout.coppafeel.org/home Here you will find a step-by-step guide and a lot of breast awareness information.

33. A Gift – Written by Lauren

When Mum asked me to write a chapter in this book, I think she thought I could offer some insights into some of the other things that have been discussed already. A 'from the child's perspective' into having breast cancer, or some more in-depth detail into some of the other things mentioned: miscarriage (I unfortunately had a molar pregnancy in 2021), or anxiety (I've unfortunately always had a problem with this one). And I was prepared to. I'm happy to talk about any, and all, of those things. Much like Mum, I have a very unlimited filter and will share my personal life openly and honestly to anyone who asks or will even bear to listen. I'll always be overtly vulnerable, show my tears, and will never hesitate to encourage others to do the same.

This book isn't about me though; it's about Mum; and so, I have decided to do this a little differently. Instead of writing about me or giving more detail into other areas in this book that have already been covered somewhat, I want to write about something that isn't in here at all. I want to write about a part of Mum that existed long before the cancer and continues to exist long after, and a part of Mum that she probably wouldn't even consider including in this book if I didn't do it myself. I'm not even sure she's always aware of how much of a blessing to me that this part of her is.

It's a part though that I have always admired and always felt inspired by: Mum's bravery and readiness to give new things a go. I can quite literally picture her in my mind right now, shaking her head vigorously back and forth, or even reading this with one eye shut so that she only has to half-digest this information, because she won't feel brave. If you are sitting next to her G, do me a favour and chuck her a pillow to hide behind. But whilst Mum thinks the challenges and illnesses she's faced makes for an interesting story, I think *she*, as a person, makes for an interesting story.

My mum doesn't want to bungee jump or go cave diving and she never will. She feels uncomfortable on planes and in crowded rooms. There are definite worries with health and family, and she has lots of insecurities. On a real level, if you ever want to see true fear in my mum's eyes, all you have to do is phone her, or even better, video call her.

But what terrifies her the most, and in turn, makes her incredibly brave, is being unhappy or settling. Mum doesn't believe that any goal or dream or insane idea is too much or too big – she's completely unhinged in the best possible way. There's always a business idea or creative idea or travel idea that's ticking over in Mum's head. Some of them surface and you get to see the result of them, some of them don't, because she's on to the next thing. It can be chaotic, overwhelming, and occasionally even stressful to be this way, and I know, because she passed it down to me.

Writing this book is one example of an idea that came to be, the original blogs being another; always wanting to try new things, live an exciting life with no regrets or questions at the end of it, and help other people along the way wherever possible. If Mum decided to be a doctor tomorrow (she won't, she can't look at needles) I'd have no doubt (other than the needle problem) that she'd actually do it.

I've watched Mum over the years train to be a hairdresser because it was something she'd wanted to do since school; Kieron and I spent our evenings after school at Nanna's whilst Mum spent her evenings at college. I've watched her start and run her own hairdressing business; working mobile in different people's houses, washing people's hair in their kitchen sinks, to then having a salon built inside our home (with a proper fancy hairdresser sink!).

I've watched Mum decide to go to university and do everything that she needed to get there and make it happen; going back to college, learning how to study and write essays for the first time in over twenty years, and travelling hours each way. I've watched her train in jobs that she has been so excited for, and then when she realised that they didn't bring her as much joy as she'd hoped or were causing her more stress or harm than anticipated, I've watched her be brave and leave. I've watched Mum manage a team and thrive, retire early, travel, buy property abroad, buy a campervan... I've learned through watching that I get to be brave and make brave decisions too, because it's all I've ever seen Mum do.

When I've decided to move away or start new careers – or quit careers to start my own businesses – she's never once questioned me or thought that I couldn't achieve my goals too. She probably believed I could more than I believed I could. She fiercely encourages without hesitation, and steps in to be the 'brave one' when I'm not feeling it myself. She's my biggest supporter, sharing my wins with me, and also being a non-judgemental sounding board when big ambitions aren't going so smoothly.

Mum gives me the permission to do something that no one else on this planet has ever given me in the same way: the permission to try, because why not? What's the worst that can happen? If you don't try, how will you ever know?

Beyond the food, house, security, and money – I think that's the biggest gift I'm grateful for, because I was raised to be honest with myself about what I want to do, who I want to be, and to never let judgement from others (or internal judgement) stop me. I was raised differently than a lot of people: I was raised to live a life that's happy, fulfilling, exciting and passionate at whatever cost; and if it's not those things, it's never too late or too shameful to change it.

So, here's a gift from her to me, and then from me to you: it's never too late to do, have or be anything that you want; stop wasting time and make it happen.

34.   An Up-to-Date Update

This January (2022) I had a severe headache, a weird cold feeling in my face, and earache, that lasted three weeks. It was arranged for me to have an early scan, at Addenbrooke's, on the alien in my head to see if there were any changes to the Epidermoid cyst that could be causing these issues. Six weeks later I had a call from the Skull Base Clinic nurse who told me that the cyst was stable (yay!) but they had found something else – of course they had! A cavernoma (also known as a cavernous angiomas/cavernous hemangiomas/cerebral cavernous malformation) is an abnormal cluster of bubbles (or caverns, hence the name) that are filled with blood – making them look like a raspberry (cool, eh?!) This is in the top right-hand part of my brain and only a couple of millimetres in size. If it bleeds it can cause problems (such as weakness to my left side, strokes, and can even be life-threatening) but there is no evidence to suggest it has so far. Guess I'll have to give this one a name as well! The consultants at Addenbrooke's aren't overly worried about this 'new' thing and they will monitor it, along with Alan the alien, on a yearly basis unless I start having more symptoms. But it has scared me, made me aware (again) that life may be short. Life seems to keep throwing curve balls (or more appropriately named – shite balls) at us and although I keep trying to live for today, not worry about tomorrow – sometimes the fear gets too much, too overwhelming, and I cry…lots! But then I try to get back to the inappropriate humour, I shake myself down, dust myself off, and book the next flight!

Since I wrote about having gone through the menopause, induced by the Zoladex injections, I have had a couple of full-blown periods that brought all the usual joys – excruciating stomach cramps, period poos, and having to wear massive, uncomfortable pads all day and night. Clearly my body is protesting and claiming I'm still too young (I wish) to go through the menopause, but come on, it's been four flipping years – I've got used to not having periods. And the worrying thing is that I thought I was coming out of the other side, with fewer hot flushes, hooray, but now I'm thinking I'll have to start the menopause, and all its wonderful symptoms, from the beginning again! My oncology team are waiting to see if I return to having a regular menstrual cycle, and if so then we will have to think of the next plan, which will be to either restart the Zoladex injections or to have a hysterectomy – fun, fun, fun!

And I'm not sure if I've mentioned it – and if I haven't you have probably gathered by now…but I don't have cancer anymore! Didn't want any spoilers to stop you turning the page, haha!

A Letter to Myself After Cancer

Dear Mel (AC),

Try not to forget to enjoy life, don't take it for granted or too seriously – tomorrow is not guaranteed for any of us. But don't be too hard on yourself if you do. It's normal to worry about the small stuff – the washing, the dodgy haircut, the muffin top (more like a three-tiered cake)! Just try not to dwell on it…be grateful that you have enough hair to have a dodgy haircut!

Don't worry about being your 'old' self – you weren't all that! Remember to always value those you love, the people who stepped up for you, those that go the extra mile.

Yes, you will want to live life to the full, but don't be afraid to say 'no' to things you really don't want to do – stop trying to please everyone all of the time.

Life will continue to throw massive challenges straight in your face, at full force. But you will cope, you will boss it, you will keep smiling/laughing/crying through it.

Go on…get out there, enjoy. Laugh, love, dance, sing, do things that make you smile, that give you joy, and even scare you a bit. Who knows what's around the corner but try not to worry – it's a waste of time and won't change anything, but may stop you having the life you want, you deserve.

Lots of love x

Terminology Cheat Sheet

So that you Know What the Hell I've Been Talking About In Simple Terms, so we can all understand…

AC – After Cancer

BC – Before Cancer

Biopsy – Take a small sample from the body to do some clever tests

Cancer – Where cells go a bit mad in the body and then cause pretty much every other thing on this list

Cannula – A not-so-fun needle that's connected to a tube, allowing all the potions and magic stuff in

Chemotherapy (Chemo) – Poison that's an amazing cancer-killer, but makes you feel incredibly poo in the process

Diagnosis – The name for whatever illness or problem my body has decided to have that particular week

ER+ – Breast cancer with Estrogen Receptors; fuelling and helping the cancer to grow (I don't really understand them but I know they're not good!!)

Fanwah – Vagina, referring to mine in most of the cases in this book

HER2+ – Breast cancer with Human Epidermal growth factor Receptor 2…. Again, all we really need to know is that it's not good (and it's also super aggressive!)

Hormone Therapy – Something I have in the form of a pill, and have to take for 10 years now that I no longer have cancer. In a nutshell, it really just stops the bastard from coming back, also yay!

HRT – Hormone Replacement Therapy: Stops the menopause from being such a pain in the arse

Lumpectomy – The operation where they removed the lump of cancer from my boob, and they do come with a warning: DO NOT pretend to be a polar bear days after this, it will NOT end well...

Mammogram – X-Rays to detect cancer done by squeezing the boob really bloody hard

Mastectomy – An operation that removes the entire boob, rather than just a lump

Menopause – When estrogen levels in women decline, made famous for the exciting news that periods stop, but lesser known for all the other crap that goes alongside it

MRI Scan – If you're clever: Magnetic Resonance Imaging; if you're less clever, like me, it's that big spaceship-looking-tube you see on TV that scans you through magnetic fields and radio waves

MUGA Scan – MUGA stands for Multigated Acquisition Scan which makes zero sense, but basically, it tests how well your heart ventricles pump

NHS – Known in some circles as the National Health Service, but for circles that have actually needed them, the National Hero Service

Oncology – The diagnosis and treatment of all the cancery stuff (and a department in the hospital)

OMG – Oh My God

Osteoporosis – Where your bones get really weak, making it a lot easier to break them – often found in the elderly, but also another fabulous side effect of cancer drugs and menopause

PET Scan – Not a scan of puppies, but a Positron Emission Tomography which looks at your tissues and organs (really not as cute as puppies)

Plastics – Plastic surgery, or the plastic surgery department – not somewhere I expected my chemo to send me

PMS – Premenstrual Syndrome is all the fun side effects of a period, before the period even arrives

Radiotherapy – Using very clever radiation to kill cancer cells, and resulting in the smallest tattoos I have (which is quite the feat considering I picked my previous two based on the fact that they were the smallest ones the shop had!)

Shingles – Chicken pox for adults. And worse

Side Effects – All the crappy extra illnesses and problems that come from taking a drug that makes you better

Terminal – A person that cannot be cured

TIA – When your brain has a bit of a wobble and has a mini-stroke

Tinnitus – An annoying buzzing or ringing inside your ears

TMI – Too Much Information

Tumour – A mass of tissue: sometimes cancer, sometimes not, but either way, it's not very friendly

Ultrasound – Using sound waves to get images of the body (how clever!)

Vertigo – Feeling like everything is spinning. It's like feeling dizzy but worse

WTF – What The Fuck

Acknowledgements

Gorgeous Graham, alias Big G, alias my long-suffering husband. Thank you for always allowing me to be free to follow whatever dream I have, at any given time! Thank you for being the best nurse ever (well apart from during poogate), you are a much better person than me. Also, thank you for being patient with me (most of the time) and worshipping the ground I walk on. I love you. Here's to many more years of adventures and growing old together.

To the most wonderful human beings, Lauren and Kieron, thank you both for loving me like you do. You have both grown into the most amazing people and I couldn't be prouder of you. Thank you for supporting me, for making me laugh when all I want to do is cry, for making me the mum I am – I am truly blessed to have you both and I love you so very much.

For my Mum and Dad. Thank you so much for being the best parents I could have wished for. You gave me everything, taught me everything, including how to love, the importance of morals and manners and have always shown me so much love and support. I will forever be grateful and feel blessed to have been chosen by you, love you loads.

To my sister, Bryony, and nephew, Connor, thank you for always being there for me. Thanks, Bry, for attending oncology appointments, for the note taking, and for the unfailing check-ins! I love you both tons.

Kerstey and Nic, thank you and I love you both. You always support me in my pipe dreams even when most of them do not come to fruition – but this one has! Thank you for always having my back and for being there for me and mine.

To those who helped me go from a rough draft to this book, with so much encouragement and support, thank you. Lauren, Caroline, Jamie, Alice, Adele, Tina, and Auntie Dot – thank you for proofreading and making so many suggestions which definitely improved the readability. Thank you for the wise and kind words, which made me feel this may actually be something people would like to read, and even find helpful hopefully.

I am so grateful for the love and support of friends, and family not already mentioned, in Felixstowe, further afield in the UK, and across the world. Thank you for the gifts, flowers, coffee dates and keeping me sane during treatment. Thank you to those who told me I should write this book. I'm not sure how it will be received but I am so grateful for the encouragement – Who knew I could write, and then publish, a book?

Thank you to the most amazing former colleagues at Otley College. Thank you all so much for the care packages, the love, support and encouragement you gave me during and after my treatment. Sorry not to name names but there are so many of you. And knowing my brain, I would leave someone out – I should have written you all down on post-it notes! But know that you all have a special place in my heart.

To the Cancer Club ladies. Even though I didn't want cancer buddies, I have made friends for life. Thank you for all of the laughter, the tears, and the ongoing support. It's good to talk to someone who can relate to what you are going through, even though all of our stories varied immensely.

Thank you seems too 'small' a statement. But thank you to Ipswich hospital and Addenbrooke's hospital for the ongoing treatment and care. Your doctors are wizards and your nurses are angels. We are so lucky in the UK to have the NHS. I am eternally grateful.

To Publishing Push. Thank you for helping me make my dream a reality…now to make it a best seller! Haha!

And finally, thank you to anyone who has taken the time to get to this point – I appreciate you and hope you have enjoyed it. Anyone who has been touched by this hideous disease, either personally or with a loved one, will have learned far more about the 'joys' of cancer than they ever wished to. Hopefully my story may have helped with some understanding, even if just a little.

Printed in Great Britain
by Amazon